2. Cottage cheese with sliced peaches

Ingredient:

- 1 cup low•fat or non•fat cottage cheese
- 1 medium peach, sliced
- Cinnamon (optional)

Instructions:

1. Rinse and slice the peach into thin slices.

2. Scoop the cottage cheese into a bowl or plate.

3. Arrange the sliced peaches on top of the cottage cheese.

4. Optionally, sprinkle a light dusting of cinnamon over the top.

This dish is perfect for post•gastric bypass patients for a few reasons:

- Cottage cheese is a great source of protein, which is important for healing and maintaining muscle mass after surgery.

- Peaches are a soft, easy•to•digest fruit that provides natural sweetness and nutrients without being too heavy on the stomach.

- The combination of protein•rich cottage cheese and the natural sugars in the peaches can help satisfy hunger and cravings.

- It's a simple, no•cook meal that requires minimal preparation, which can be helpful when appetite and energy levels are low after surgery.

You can adjust the portion sizes as needed to meet your individual nutritional needs. This makes for a quick, healthy, and satisfying post•op snack or light meal. Enjoy!

3. Greek yogurt with berries

Ingredient:

• 1 cup plain Greek yogurt (low•fat or non•fat)
• 1/2 cup mixed berries (such as blueberries, raspberries, blackberries)
• 1 tsp honey (optional)

Instructions:

1. Scoop the Greek yogurt into a bowl or container.

2. Gently fold in the mixed berries.

3. If desired, drizzle 1 tsp of honey over the top.

This simple dish is an excellent choice for post•gastric bypass patients for several reasons:

• Greek yogurt is high in protein, which is crucial for healing, maintaining muscle mass, and feeling full after surgery.

• Berries are a great source of fiber, vitamins, and antioxidants. The soft texture and natural sweetness make them easy to digest.

• The combination of protein•rich yogurt and fiber•filled berries creates a nutrient•dense snack or light meal that can help manage hunger and cravings.

• The honey (if used) provides a touch of natural sweetness without adding too many calories or carbs.

You can adjust the portion sizes as needed to meet your individual nutritional requirements. This dish is quick and easy to prepare, making it a convenient option when energy levels are low after surgery.

Feel free to experiment with different types of berries or even try other fresh fruit like sliced peaches or mango. The key is to focus on foods that are high in protein, fiber, and nutrients while being gentle on the digestive system.

Congratulations on taking a monumental step towards a healthier, more vibrant life through gastric bypass surgery! This transformative procedure is just the beginning of your journey. What comes next is equally crucial: adopting a nutritious, balanced diet that supports your new lifestyle and ensures long-term success.

Why This Cookbook?
"The Post-Gastric Bypass Cookbook: 110+ Nutritious Recipes for Post-Gastric Bypass Success" is designed with your unique needs in mind. After gastric bypass surgery, your body undergoes significant changes that require a specialized approach to nutrition. This cookbook is here to guide you through this new chapter, providing delicious, easy-to-follow recipes that are perfectly suited to your dietary requirements.

What You'll Find Inside
- *Nutrient-Dense Recipes:* Every recipe in this book is crafted to maximize nutrition while minimizing calories, ensuring you get the essential vitamins and minerals needed for your recovery and long-term health.

- *Variety and Flavor:* Eating well after surgery doesn't mean sacrificing taste. Enjoy a diverse range of meals, from hearty breakfasts to satisfying dinners and everything in between.

- *Step-by-Step Guidance:* Whether you're an experienced cook or a kitchen novice, our clear instructions and helpful tips make meal preparation simple and stress-free.

- *Portion Control:* Learn how to manage portion sizes effectively, helping you avoid overeating and maintain your weight loss goals.

- *Post-Surgery Stages:* Find recipes tailored to each phase of your post-surgery diet, from the initial liquid stage to more advanced solid foods.

Your Path to Success
Adapting to a new way of eating can be challenging, but with the right tools and knowledge, it becomes an exciting adventure. This cookbook is more than just a collection of recipes; it's a companion on your journey to a healthier you. By embracing these nutritious meals, you'll not only support your weight loss but also enhance your overall well-being.

Remember, every step you take towards better nutrition is a step towards a healthier, happier life. Welcome to "The Post-Gastric Bypass Cookbook: 110+ Nutritious Recipes for Post-Gastric Bypass Success." Let's embark on this culinary journey together and celebrate each milestone along the way. Happy cooking!

1. Scrambled eggs with spinach

Ingredient:

- 6 eggs
- 2 tbsp milk or water
- 1 tsp butter or olive oil
- 2 cups fresh spinach, chopped
- 1 clove garlic, minced
- Salt and pepper to taste

Instructions:

1. In a bowl, whisk together the eggs and milk/water until well combined. Season with a pinch of salt and pepper.

2. In a nonstick skillet, melt the butter or heat the olive oil over medium heat.

3. Add the minced garlic and sauté for 1 minute until fragrant.

4. Add the chopped spinach and cook for 2•3 minutes, stirring frequently, until the spinach is wilted.

5. Pour in the egg mixture and use a spatula to gently push and fold the eggs as they cook, about 2•3 minutes, until the eggs are softly scrambled.

6. Remove from heat and serve immediately. Enjoy your scrambled eggs with fresh spinach!

You can adjust the amount of spinach to your preference. The garlic adds nice flavor, but you can omit it if desired. Serve with toast, potatoes, or on its own for a healthy breakfast.

4. Smoothie with protein powder, almond milk, and banana

Ingredient:

- 1 cup unsweetened almond milk
- 1 scoop vanilla or unflavored protein powder
- 1 medium banana, frozen
- 1 tbsp almond butter (optional)

Instructions:

1. Add the almond milk and protein powder to a blender. Blend until smooth.

2. Add the frozen banana and almond butter (if using). Blend again until well combined and creamy.

This smoothie is an excellent choice for post•gastric bypass patients for several reasons:

Protein: The protein powder provides a concentrated source of high•quality protein, which is essential for healing, maintaining muscle mass, and feeling full after surgery.

Almond milk: Unsweetened almond milk is low in calories and carbs, yet still provides healthy fats and nutrients. It's gentle on the digestive system.

Banana: Frozen bananas add natural sweetness, fiber, and potassium without being too heavy. The soft texture is easy to digest.

Almond butter (optional): Provides additional healthy fats and protein to help keep you satisfied.

This smoothie is quick and easy to prepare, making it a convenient option when you may have limited energy or appetite after surgery. You can adjust the amounts of each ingredient to suit your individual needs and preferences.

Some other variations could include:
- Adding a handful of spinach or kale for extra nutrients
- Using Greek yogurt instead of almond milk for more protein
- Swapping the banana for other soft fruits like berries or mango

The key is to focus on nutrient•dense, easy•to•digest ingredients that will provide the nourishment your body needs during the recovery process.

5. Hard•boiled eggs

Ingredient:

• Eggs

Instructions:

1. Place the eggs in a single layer in a saucepan and cover with cold water by 1 inch.

2. Bring the water to a boil over high heat. Once the water reaches a full boil, remove the pan from the heat and cover.

3. Let the eggs sit in the hot water for the following times:
• Soft•boiled: 3•5 minutes
• Hard•boiled: 12 minutes

4. Drain the hot water and cover the eggs with cold water to stop the cooking.

5. Let the eggs sit in the cold water for 5 minutes.

6. Peel the eggs and enjoy! The yolks should be fully cooked and set for hard•boiled eggs.

Tips:
• Older eggs peel more easily than very fresh eggs.
• Adding a teaspoon of baking soda to the water can also help with peeling.
• Hard•boiled eggs in the shell can be stored in the refrigerator for up to 1 week.

6. Tuna salad with light mayo and celery

Ingredient:

- 2 (5 oz) cans tuna, drained
- 2•3 tbsp light mayonnaise
- 1/4 cup diced celery
- 1 tbsp diced onion (optional)
- 1 tsp Dijon mustard
- Salt and pepper to taste

Instructions:

1. In a medium bowl, combine the drained tuna, light mayonnaise, diced celery, and onion (if using).

2. Mix well until all the ingredients are evenly distributed.

3. Stir in the Dijon mustard and season with salt and pepper to taste.

Tips for Post•Gastric Bypass:

- Use light or low•fat mayonnaise to keep the calories and fat low.

- Limit the amount of mayonnaise used • just enough to lightly coat the tuna.

- Include plenty of crunchy vegetables like celery to add fiber and volume without a lot of calories.

- Avoid adding too many high•calorie mix•ins like cheese, nuts, or dried fruit.

- Serve the tuna salad on a bed of greens, with whole grain crackers, or stuffed into a tomato.

This tuna salad provides lean protein from the tuna, fiber from the celery, and healthy fats from the light mayo. It's a nutritious and satisfying option for those following a post•gastric bypass diet.

7. Grilled chicken breast with steamed broccoli

Ingredient:

• 4 boneless, skinless chicken breasts (about 4•6 oz each)
• 1 tbsp olive oil
• Salt and pepper to taste
• 1 lb broccoli florets

Instructions:

1. Preheat grill or grill pan to medium•high heat.

2. Brush the chicken breasts lightly with olive oil and season with salt and pepper.

3. Grill the chicken for 4•6 minutes per side, until cooked through and no longer pink in the center. The internal temperature should reach 165°F.

4. While the chicken is grilling, steam the broccoli florets until tender•crisp, about 5•7 minutes.

5. Serve the grilled chicken breast alongside the steamed broccoli.

Tips for Post•Gastric Bypass:

• Chicken breast is an excellent lean protein source that is easy to digest after surgery.

• Steamed broccoli provides fiber, vitamins, and minerals without a lot of calories or fat.

• Keep portion sizes modest • aim for 4•6 oz of chicken and 1/2 to 1 cup of broccoli.

• Avoid heavy sauces or gravies, which can be high in calories and fat.

• Season simply with herbs, spices, lemon juice, or a small amount of low•fat dressing.

• Drink water or unsweetened beverages with the meal to stay hydrated.

This grilled chicken and steamed broccoli dish is a nutritious, balanced, and easy•to•digest meal that supports the nutritional needs of those following a post•gastric bypass diet.

8. Baked fish with lemon and herbs

Ingredient:

• 4 (4•6 oz) white fish fillets (such as tilapia, cod, or halibut)
• 2 tbsp fresh lemon juice
• 1 tbsp olive oil
• 1 tsp dried oregano
• 1 tsp dried basil
• Salt and pepper to taste
• Lemon wedges for serving

Instructions:

1. Preheat the oven to 400°F. Lightly grease a baking dish or line with parchment paper.

2. Place the fish fillets in the prepared baking dish. Drizzle with the lemon juice and olive oil, making sure to coat the fish evenly.

3. Sprinkle the dried oregano and basil over the top of the fish. Season with salt and pepper.

4. Bake for 12•15 minutes, or until the fish is opaque and flakes easily with a fork.

5. Serve the baked fish immediately, with lemon wedges on the side.

Tips for Post•Gastric Bypass:

• White fish is an excellent lean protein source that is easy to digest after surgery.

• Lemon and herbs add flavor without the need for heavy sauces or butter.

• Baking the fish keeps it moist and tender without added fat.

• Portion sizes should be kept modest, around 4•6 oz of fish per serving.

• Pair the fish with steamed vegetables or a small salad for a complete, balanced meal.

• Drink water or unsweetened beverages with the meal to stay hydrated.

This baked fish dish is a simple, flavorful, and nutritious option that supports the dietary needs of those following a post•gastric bypass diet.

9. Turkey meatballs with tomato sauce

Ingredient:

- 1 lb ground turkey
- 1/4 cup whole wheat breadcrumbs
- 1 egg, lightly beaten
- 2 tbsp grated Parmesan cheese
- 2 cloves garlic, minced
- 1 tsp dried oregano
- 1/2 tsp salt
- 1/4 tsp black pepper
- 1 (15 oz) can no•sugar•added tomato sauce
- 2 tbsp fresh basil, chopped (optional)

Instructions:

1. Preheat the oven to 400°F. Line a baking sheet with parchment paper.

2. In a medium bowl, combine the ground turkey, breadcrumbs, egg, Parmesan, garlic, oregano, salt, and pepper. Mix well until all the ingredients are evenly distributed.

3. Roll the mixture into 1•inch meatballs and place them on the prepared baking sheet.

4. Bake the meatballs for 18•20 minutes, or until they are cooked through and no longer pink in the center.

5. In a saucepan, heat the tomato sauce over medium heat until warmed through.

6. Gently add the cooked meatballs to the tomato sauce and stir to coat.

7. Serve the turkey meatballs with the tomato sauce, garnished with fresh basil if desired.

Tips for Post•Gastric Bypass:

- Ground turkey is a lean protein that is easy to digest after surgery.
- Whole wheat breadcrumbs provide fiber and complex carbohydrates.
- The portion size of 1•inch meatballs is appropriate for post•gastric bypass.
- Tomato sauce is a low•calorie, nutrient•dense sauce that complements the meatballs.
- Avoid heavy, creamy sauces that can be difficult to digest.
- Serve with a side of steamed vegetables for a complete, balanced meal.

This turkey meatball dish is a flavorful, nutritious, and easy•to•digest option for those following a post•gastric bypass diet.

10. Lentil soup

Ingredient:

- 1 tbsp olive oil
- 1 onion, diced
- 2 carrots, peeled and diced
- 2 celery stalks, diced
- 3 garlic cloves, minced
- 1 cup dried brown or green lentils, rinsed
- 4 cups low·sodium chicken or vegetable broth
- 1 (14.5 oz) can diced tomatoes
- 1 tsp dried thyme
- 1 tsp dried oregano
- Salt and pepper to taste
- Fresh parsley, chopped (for garnish)

Instructions:

1. In a large pot or Dutch oven, heat the olive oil over medium heat. Add the onion, carrots, and celery. Sauté for 5·7 minutes, until the vegetables are softened.

2. Add the garlic and sauté for 1 minute more, until fragrant.

3. Stir in the lentils, broth, diced tomatoes, thyme, and oregano. Season with salt and pepper to taste.

4. Bring the soup to a boil, then reduce the heat and let it simmer for 20·25 minutes, or until the lentils are tender.

5. Ladle the lentil soup into bowls and garnish with fresh chopped parsley, if desired.

Tips for Post·Gastric Bypass:

- Lentils are an excellent source of lean protein and fiber, which are important for post·surgery nutrition.
- The broth·based soup is easy to digest and won't overwhelm the stomach.
- Vegetables like carrots, celery, and onions add nutrients and texture without a lot of calories.
- Portion sizes should be kept modest, around 1 cup of soup per serving.
- Avoid adding heavy cream or cheese, which can be difficult to digest.
- Drink water or unsweetened beverages with the soup to stay hydrated.

11. Black bean soup

Ingredient:

- 1 tbsp olive oil
- 1 onion, diced
- 2 carrots, peeled and diced
- 2 celery stalks, diced
- 3 garlic cloves, minced
- 2 (15 oz) cans black beans, rinsed and drained
- 4 cups low•sodium chicken or vegetable broth
- 1 tsp ground cumin
- 1 tsp dried oregano
- 1/2 tsp smoked paprika
- Salt and pepper to taste
- Chopped cilantro for garnish (optional)

Instructions:

1. In a large pot or Dutch oven, heat the olive oil over medium heat. Add the onion, carrots, and celery. Sauté for 5•7 minutes, until the vegetables are softened.

2. Add the garlic and sauté for 1 minute more, until fragrant.

3. Stir in the black beans, broth, cumin, oregano, and smoked paprika. Season with salt and pepper to taste.

4. Bring the soup to a boil, then reduce the heat and let it simmer for 15•20 minutes, allowing the flavors to meld.

5. Using an immersion blender or regular blender, puree about half of the soup to create a creamy texture, leaving the other half chunky.

6. Ladle the black bean soup into bowls and garnish with chopped cilantro, if desired.

Tips for Post•Gastric Bypass:

- Black beans are an excellent source of lean protein and fiber, which are important for post•surgery nutrition.
- The broth•based soup is easy to digest and won't overwhelm the stomach.
- Vegetables like carrots, celery, and onions add nutrients and texture without a lot of calories.
- Portion sizes should be kept modest, around 1 cup of soup per serving.

12. Minestrone soup (with small pasta)

Ingredient:

• 1 tbsp olive oil
• 1 onion, diced
• 2 carrots, peeled and diced
• 2 celery stalks, diced
• 3 garlic cloves, minced
• 1 (15 oz) can diced tomatoes
• 4 cups low•sodium chicken or vegetable broth
• 1 (15 oz) can kidney beans, rinsed and drained
• 1 cup small pasta (such as ditalini or small shells)
• 1 tsp dried oregano
• 1 tsp dried basil
• Salt and pepper to taste
• Grated Parmesan cheese for serving (optional)

Instructions:

1. In a large pot or Dutch oven, heat the olive oil over medium heat. Add the onion, carrots, and celery. Sauté for 5•7 minutes, until the vegetables are softened.

2. Add the garlic and sauté for 1 minute more, until fragrant.

3. Stir in the diced tomatoes, broth, kidney beans, small pasta, oregano, and basil. Season with salt and pepper to taste.

4. Bring the soup to a boil, then reduce the heat and let it simmer for 15•20 minutes, or until the pasta is tender.

5. Ladle the minestrone soup into bowls and serve with a sprinkle of grated Parmesan cheese, if desired.

Tips for Post•Gastric Bypass:

• The small pasta provides a source of complex carbohydrates in a manageable portion size.
• Kidney beans are a good source of lean protein and fiber, which are important for post•surgery nutrition.
• Vegetables like carrots, celery, and onions add nutrients and texture without a lot of calories.
• The broth•based soup is easy to digest and won't overwhelm the stomach.

13. Chicken noodle soup (with small noodles)

Ingredient:

- 1 tbsp olive oil
- 1 onion, diced
- 2 carrots, peeled and diced
- 2 celery stalks, diced
- 3 garlic cloves, minced
- 4 cups low•sodium chicken broth
- 2 cups shredded cooked chicken
- 1 cup small pasta or noodles (such as ditalini, orzo, or mini farfalle)
- 1 tsp dried thyme
- 1 tsp dried parsley
- Salt and pepper to taste
- Chopped fresh parsley for garnish (optional)

Instructions:

1. In a large pot or Dutch oven, heat the olive oil over medium heat. Add the onion, carrots, and celery. Sauté for 5•7 minutes, until the vegetables are softened.

2. Add the garlic and sauté for 1 minute more, until fragrant.

3. Pour in the chicken broth and bring the soup to a boil.

4. Stir in the shredded cooked chicken, small pasta or noodles, thyme, and dried parsley. Season with salt and pepper to taste.

5. Reduce the heat and let the soup simmer for 10•15 minutes, or until the pasta or noodles are tender.

6. Ladle the chicken noodle soup into bowls and garnish with chopped fresh parsley, if desired.

Tips for Post•Gastric Bypass:

- Chicken is a lean protein that is easy to digest after surgery.
- The small pasta or noodles provide a source of complex carbohydrates in a manageable portion size.
- Vegetables like carrots, celery, and onions add nutrients and texture without a lot of calories.
- The broth•based soup is easy to digest and won't overwhelm the stomach.

14. Butternut squash soup

Ingredient:

- 1 tbsp olive oil
- 1 onion, diced
- 2 carrots, peeled and diced
- 2 celery stalks, diced
- 3 garlic cloves, minced
- 1 (3 lb) butternut squash, peeled, seeded, and cubed
- 4 cups low•sodium chicken or vegetable broth
- 1 tsp ground cumin
- 1/2 tsp ground cinnamon
- Salt and pepper to taste
- Chopped fresh parsley for garnish (optional)

Instructions:

1. In a large pot or Dutch oven, heat the olive oil over medium heat. Add the onion, carrots, and celery. Sauté for 5•7 minutes, until the vegetables are softened.

2. Add the garlic and sauté for 1 minute more, until fragrant.

3. Stir in the cubed butternut squash, broth, cumin, and cinnamon. Season with salt and pepper to taste.

4. Bring the soup to a boil, then reduce the heat and let it simmer for 20•25 minutes, or until the squash is very soft.

5. Using an immersion blender or regular blender, puree the soup until smooth and creamy.

6. Ladle the butternut squash soup into bowls and garnish with chopped fresh parsley, if desired.

Tips for Post•Gastric Bypass:

- Butternut squash is a nutrient•dense vegetable that is high in fiber and vitamins, which are important for post•surgery nutrition.
- The creamy texture of the pureed soup is easy to digest and won't overwhelm the stomach.

This butternut squash soup is a comforting, nutritious, and easy•to•digest option for those following a post•gastric bypass diet.

15. Cream of mushroom soup (made with low•fat milk)

Ingredient:

- 1 tbsp olive oil
- 1 onion, diced
- 8 oz mushrooms, sliced
- 2 garlic cloves, minced
- 2 tbsp all•purpose flour
- 2 cups low•fat milk
- 2 cups low•sodium chicken or vegetable broth
- 1 tsp dried thyme
- Salt and pepper to taste
- Chopped fresh parsley for garnish (optional)

Instructions:

1. In a large pot or Dutch oven, heat the olive oil over medium heat. Add the onion and sauté for 3•4 minutes, until translucent.

2. Add the sliced mushrooms and garlic. Sauté for 5•7 minutes, until the mushrooms are softened.

3. Sprinkle the flour over the mushroom mixture and stir to coat. Cook for 1 minute.

4. Gradually whisk in the low•fat milk and broth. Bring the soup to a simmer and cook for 10•15 minutes, stirring occasionally, until thickened.

5. Stir in the dried thyme and season with salt and pepper to taste.

6. Using an immersion blender or regular blender, puree the soup until smooth and creamy.

7. Ladle the cream of mushroom soup into bowls and garnish with chopped fresh parsley, if desired.

Tips for Post•Gastric Bypass:

- Using low•fat milk instead of heavy cream keeps the soup lower in calories and fat, which can be easier to digest.
- The pureed texture of the soup is gentle on the stomach after surgery.
- Mushrooms provide a savory, umami flavor without a lot of calories.

16. Hummus with baby carrots

Ingredient:

• 1 (15 oz) can chickpeas (garbanzo beans), rinsed and drained
• 2 tbsp tahini (sesame seed paste)
• 2 tbsp fresh lemon juice
• 1 garlic clove, minced
• 2 tbsp olive oil
• 1/4 tsp ground cumin
• 1/4 tsp paprika
• Salt and pepper to taste
• 1 lb baby carrots, washed and trimmed

Instructions:

1. In a food processor or high•powered blender, combine the chickpeas, tahini, lemon juice, garlic, olive oil, cumin, and paprika. Blend until smooth and creamy, scraping down the sides as needed.

2. Season the hummus with salt and pepper to taste.

3. Transfer the hummus to a serving bowl or plate.

4. Arrange the baby carrots around the hummus, making it easy for dipping.

Tips for Post•Gastric Bypass:

• Chickpeas are a great source of lean protein and fiber, which are important for post•surgery nutrition.
• Tahini provides healthy fats from sesame seeds, which can help with nutrient absorption.
• The crunchy texture of the baby carrots provides a satisfying contrast to the creamy hummus.
• Portion sizes should be kept modest, around 2•3 tbsp of hummus and 4•6 baby carrots per serving.
• Avoid pairing the hummus with high•fat or high•carb dippers like pita bread or chips.
• Drink water or unsweetened beverages with the snack to stay hydrated.

This hummus and baby carrot combination is a nutritious, easy•to•digest, and satisfying snack or light meal for those following a post•gastric bypass diet.

17. Guacamole with sliced bell peppers

Ingredient:

- 2 ripe avocados, pitted and mashed
- 2 tbsp fresh lime juice
- 2 tbsp diced onion
- 1 garlic clove, minced
- 2 tbsp chopped cilantro (optional)
- 1/4 tsp ground cumin
- Salt and pepper to taste
- 1 red bell pepper, sliced into strips
- 1 yellow bell pepper, sliced into strips

Instructions:

1. In a medium bowl, mash the avocados with a fork or potato masher.

2. Stir in the lime juice, onion, garlic, cilantro (if using), and cumin. Season with salt and pepper to taste.

3. Mix the ingredients together until well combined.

4. Arrange the sliced bell pepper strips around the guacamole, making it easy for dipping.

Tips for Post•Gastric Bypass:

• Avocados are a great source of healthy fats, which can help with nutrient absorption after surgery.

• The crunchy texture of the bell peppers provides a satisfying contrast to the creamy guacamole.

• Portion sizes should be kept modest, around 2•3 tbsp of guacamole and 4•6 bell pepper strips per serving.

• Avoid pairing the guacamole with high•carb dippers like tortilla chips or pita bread. Drink water or unsweetened beverages with the snack to stay hydrated.

This guacamole and bell pepper combination is a nutritious, easy•to•digest, and satisfying snack or light meal for those following a post•gastric bypass diet.

18. Baba ganoush with cucumber slices

Ingredient:

- 1 medium eggplant
- 2 tbsp tahini (sesame seed paste)
- 2 tbsp fresh lemon juice
- 1 garlic clove, minced
- 2 tbsp olive oil
- 1/4 tsp ground cumin
- Salt and pepper to taste
- 1 English cucumber, sliced

Instructions:

1. Preheat the oven to 400°F. Pierce the eggplant several times with a fork and place it on a baking sheet. Roast for 30•40 minutes, or until very soft. Allow the eggplant to cool slightly.

2. Cut the eggplant in half lengthwise and scoop out the flesh into a food processor or high•powered blender. Discard the skin.

3. Add the tahini, lemon juice, garlic, olive oil, and cumin to the eggplant. Blend until smooth and creamy, scraping down the sides as needed.

4. Season the baba ganoush with salt and pepper to taste.

5. Transfer the baba ganoush to a serving bowl or plate. Arrange the sliced cucumber around the dip, making it easy for dipping.

Tips for Post•Gastric Bypass:

- Eggplant is a low•calorie, nutrient•dense vegetable that is easy to digest after surgery.
- Tahini provides healthy fats from sesame seeds, which can help with nutrient absorption.
- The crunchy texture of the cucumber slices provides a satisfying contrast to the creamy baba ganoush.
- Portion sizes should be kept modest, around 2•3 tbsp of baba ganoush and 4•6 cucumber slices per serving.
- Avoid pairing the baba ganoush with high•carb dippers like pita bread or chips.
- Drink water or unsweetened beverages with the snack to stay hydrated.

19. Chicken salad with light mayo and grapes

Ingredient:

- 2 cups cooked, shredded chicken breast
- 2•3 tbsp light mayonnaise
- 1/4 cup diced celery
- 1/4 cup halved red grapes
- 1 tbsp chopped fresh parsley
- 1 tsp Dijon mustard
- Salt and pepper to taste

Instructions:

1. In a medium bowl, combine the shredded chicken, light mayonnaise, diced celery, halved grapes, chopped parsley, and Dijon mustard.

2. Mix all the ingredients together until well combined.. Season the chicken salad with salt and pepper to taste.

Serving Suggestions:
- Serve the chicken salad on a bed of mixed greens or spinach.
- Scoop the chicken salad into halved tomatoes or cucumber cups.
- Enjoy the chicken salad with a side of sliced cucumber or bell pepper strips.

Tips for Post•Gastric Bypass:

- Chicken breast is a lean protein that is easy to digest after surgery.
- Light mayonnaise helps keep the calories and fat content lower compared to regular mayonnaise.
- Grapes add a touch of sweetness and provide some natural sugars, which can be helpful for those with a reduced appetite.
- Celery and parsley add crunch and fresh flavor without a lot of calories.
- Portion sizes should be kept modest, around 1/2 to 1 cup of chicken salad per serving.
- Avoid pairing the chicken salad with high•carb breads or crackers.
- Drink water or unsweetened beverages with the meal to stay hydrated.

This chicken salad with light mayo and grapes is a nutritious, flavorful, and easy•to•digest option for those following a post•gastric bypass diet.

20. Egg salad with light mayo and chopped celery

Ingredient:

- 6 hard•boiled eggs, peeled and chopped
- 2•3 tbsp light mayonnaise
- 2 tbsp diced celery
- 1 tsp Dijon mustard
- 1 tbsp chopped fresh parsley (optional)
- Salt and pepper to taste

Instructions:

1. In a medium bowl, combine the chopped hard•boiled eggs, light mayonnaise, diced celery, Dijon mustard, and chopped parsley (if using).

2. Stir the ingredients together until well mixed.

3. Season the egg salad with salt and pepper to taste.

Serving Suggestions:

- Serve the egg salad on a bed of mixed greens or spinach.

- Scoop the egg salad into halved tomatoes or cucumber cups.

- Enjoy the egg salad with a side of sliced cucumber or bell pepper strips.

Tips for Post•Gastric Bypass:

- Eggs are an excellent source of lean protein that is easy to digest after surgery.

- Light mayonnaise helps keep the calories and fat content lower compared to regular mayonnaise.

- Celery adds a crunchy texture and some additional fiber without a lot of calories.

- Portion sizes should be kept modest, around 1/2 to 1 cup of egg salad per serving.

- Avoid pairing the egg salad with high•carb breads or crackers.

- Drink water or unsweetened beverages with the meal to stay hydrated.

This egg salad with light mayo and celery is a nutritious, flavorful, and easy•to•digest option for those following a post•gastric bypass diet.

21. Shrimp cocktail with sugar•free cocktail sauce

Ingredient:

For the Shrimp:
• 1 lb cooked, peeled, and deveined shrimp, chilled
• Lemon wedges for serving

For the Sugar•Free Cocktail Sauce:
• 1/2 cup no•sugar•added ketchup
• 2 tbsp prepared horseradish
• 1 tbsp fresh lemon juice
• 1 tsp Worcestershire sauce
• 1/4 tsp hot sauce (optional)
• Salt and pepper to taste

Instructions:

1. Make the cocktail sauce: In a small bowl, combine the no•sugar•added ketchup, horseradish, lemon juice, Worcestershire sauce, and hot sauce (if using). Stir well and season with salt and pepper to taste.

2. Arrange the chilled shrimp on a serving platter or in individual cocktail glasses.

3. Serve the shrimp with the sugar•free cocktail sauce and lemon wedges on the side.

Tips for Post•Gastric Bypass:

• Shrimp is a lean protein that is easy to digest after surgery.

• The sugar•free cocktail sauce provides flavor without the added sugar, which can be difficult to tolerate after gastric bypass.

• Portion sizes should be kept modest, around 4•6 shrimp and 2•3 tbsp of sauce per serving.

• Avoid pairing the shrimp cocktail with high•carb crackers or bread.

• Drink water or unsweetened beverages with the meal to stay hydrated.

This shrimp cocktail with sugar•free cocktail sauce is a light, flavorful, and easy•to•digest option for those following a post•gastric bypass diet.

22. Caprese salad (mozzarella, tomatoes, and basil)

Ingredient:

• 8 oz fresh mozzarella cheese, sliced
• 2 cups cherry or grape tomatoes, halved
• 1/4 cup fresh basil leaves, torn or chopped
• 1 tbsp balsamic glaze or reduced•calorie balsamic vinaigrette
• Salt and pepper to taste

Instructions:

1. Arrange the sliced mozzarella cheese and halved tomatoes on a serving plate or platter.

2. Sprinkle the torn or chopped fresh basil leaves over the top.

3. Drizzle the balsamic glaze or reduced•calorie balsamic vinaigrette over the salad.

4. Season with salt and pepper to taste.

Tips for Post•Gastric Bypass:

• Fresh mozzarella cheese is a good source of protein that is easy to digest after surgery.

• Tomatoes provide vitamins, minerals, and antioxidants without a lot of calories.

• Fresh basil adds flavor without the need for heavy dressings or sauces.

• The balsamic glaze or vinaigrette provides a touch of acidity and sweetness without a lot of added sugar.

• Portion sizes should be kept modest, around 1/2 to 1 cup of the salad per serving.

• Avoid pairing the caprese salad with high•carb breads or crackers.

• Drink water or unsweetened beverages with the meal to stay hydrated.

This caprese salad is a light, refreshing, and easy•to•digest option for those following a post•gastric bypass diet.

23. Cobb salad (with chicken, hard•boiled egg, and light dressing)

Ingredient:

- 5 oz mixed greens (such as romaine, spinach, and arugula)
- 4 oz grilled or roasted chicken breast, diced
- 1 hard•boiled egg, chopped
- 1/4 cup diced tomatoes
- 2 tbsp diced avocado
- 2 tbsp crumbled low•fat feta cheese
- 2 tbsp light balsamic vinaigrette or ranch dressing

Instructions:

1. In a large salad bowl, arrange the mixed greens as the base.

2. Top the greens with the diced chicken, chopped hard•boiled egg, diced tomatoes, diced avocado, and crumbled feta cheese.

3. Drizzle the light balsamic vinaigrette or ranch dressing over the salad.

4. Toss the salad gently to combine all the ingredients.

Tips for Post•Gastric Bypass:

- Chicken and hard•boiled egg provide lean protein that is easy to digest after surgery.

- Avocado and feta cheese add healthy fats and flavor without a lot of calories.

- The light dressing keeps the salad low in calories and easy to tolerate.

- Portion sizes should be kept modest, around 1 to 1.5 cups of the salad per serving.

- Avoid adding high•carb toppings like croutons or fried onions.

- Drink water or unsweetened beverages with the salad to stay hydrated.

This Cobb salad is a nutritious, filling, and easy•to•digest option for those following a post•gastric bypass diet.

24. Greek salad (with feta, olives, and light dressing)

Ingredient:

- 5 oz mixed greens (such as romaine, spinach, and arugula)
- 1/2 cup diced cucumber
- 1/4 cup diced tomatoes
- 2 tbsp crumbled low•fat feta cheese
- 2 tbsp sliced black or kalamata olives
- 1 tbsp red onion, thinly sliced
- 2 tbsp light Greek or Mediterranean•style dressing

Instructions:

1. In a large salad bowl, combine the mixed greens, diced cucumber, diced tomatoes, crumbled feta cheese, sliced olives, and thinly sliced red onion.

2. Drizzle the light Greek or Mediterranean•style dressing over the salad.

3. Toss the salad gently to coat the ingredients with the dressing.

Tips for Post•Gastric Bypass:

- The mixed greens provide a nutrient•dense base for the salad.

- Cucumber and tomatoes add crunch and hydration without a lot of calories.

- Feta cheese provides a source of protein and healthy fats that are easy to digest.

- Olives and onion add flavor without the need for heavy dressings.

- The light dressing keeps the salad low in calories and easy to tolerate.

- Portion sizes should be kept modest, around 1 to 1.5 cups of the salad per serving. Avoid adding high•carb toppings like pita bread or croutons.

- Drink water or unsweetened beverages with the salad to stay hydrated.

This Greek salad is a refreshing, flavorful, and easy•to•digest option for those following a post•gastric bypass diet.

25. Quinoa salad with vegetables

Ingredient:

• 1 cup cooked quinoa, cooled
• 1/2 cup diced cucumber
• 1/2 cup diced tomatoes
• 1/4 cup diced red onion
• 1/4 cup diced bell pepper
• 2 tbsp chopped fresh parsley
• 1 tbsp olive oil
• 1 tbsp lemon juice
• 1 tsp Dijon mustard
• Salt and pepper to taste

Instructions:

1. In a large bowl, combine the cooked and cooled quinoa, diced cucumber, tomatoes, red onion, bell pepper, and chopped parsley.

2. In a small bowl, whisk together the olive oil, lemon juice, and Dijon mustard.

3. Pour the dressing over the quinoa and vegetable mixture and toss gently to coat.

4. Season the quinoa salad with salt and pepper to taste.

Tips for Post•Gastric Bypass:

• Quinoa is a gluten•free, high•protein grain that is easy to digest after surgery.
• The vegetables provide fiber, vitamins, and minerals without a lot of calories.
• The simple dressing of olive oil, lemon juice, and Dijon mustard adds flavor without being heavy or creamy.
• Portion sizes should be kept modest, around 1/2 to 1 cup of the quinoa salad per serving.
• Avoid adding high•fat or high•calorie toppings like cheese, nuts, or dried fruit.
• Drink water or unsweetened beverages with the salad to stay hydrated.

This quinoa salad with vegetables is a nutritious, filling, and easy•to•digest option for those following a post•gastric bypass diet.

26. Tabouli salad

Ingredient:

- 1 cup cooked and cooled bulgur wheat
- 1 cup chopped fresh parsley
- 1/2 cup diced tomatoes
- 1/4 cup diced cucumber
- 2 tbsp diced red onion
- 2 tbsp fresh lemon juice
- 1 tbsp olive oil
- 1 garlic clove, minced
- Salt and pepper to taste

Instructions:

1. In a large bowl, combine the cooked and cooled bulgur wheat, chopped parsley, diced tomatoes, diced cucumber, and diced red onion.

2. In a small bowl, whisk together the lemon juice, olive oil, and minced garlic.

3. Pour the dressing over the tabouli salad and toss gently to coat the ingredients.

4. Season the tabouli salad with salt and pepper to taste.

5. Cover and refrigerate the salad for at least 30 minutes to allow the flavors to meld.

Tips for Post•Gastric Bypass:

- Bulgur wheat is a whole grain that is high in fiber and easy to digest after surgery.
- The fresh parsley, tomatoes, and cucumber provide vitamins, minerals, and hydration without a lot of calories.
- The simple lemon juice and olive oil dressing adds flavor without being heavy or creamy.
- Portion sizes should be kept modest, around 1/2 to 1 cup of the tabouli salad per serving.
- Avoid adding high•fat or high•calorie toppings like cheese or nuts.
- Drink water or unsweetened beverages with the salad to stay hydrated.

This tabouli salad is a refreshing, nutritious, and easy•to•digest option for those following a post•gastric bypass diet.

27. Three•bean salad

Ingredient:

- 1 (15 oz) can kidney beans, rinsed and drained
- 1 (15 oz) can garbanzo beans (chickpeas), rinsed and drained
- 1 (15 oz) can green beans, rinsed and drained
- 1/4 cup diced red onion
- 2 tbsp apple cider vinegar
- 1 tbsp olive oil
- 1 tsp Dijon mustard
- 1 tsp dried oregano
- Salt and pepper to taste

Instructions:

1. In a large bowl, combine the rinsed and drained kidney beans, garbanzo beans, and green beans.

2. Add the diced red onion to the bean mixture.

3. In a small bowl, whisk together the apple cider vinegar, olive oil, Dijon mustard, and dried oregano.

4. Pour the dressing over the bean salad and toss gently to coat.

5. Season the three•bean salad with salt and pepper to taste.

6. Cover and refrigerate the salad for at least 30 minutes to allow the flavors to meld.

Tips for Post•Gastric Bypass:

- The combination of kidney beans, garbanzo beans, and green beans provides a good source of lean protein and fiber, which are important for post•surgery nutrition.
- The simple vinegar•based dressing adds flavor without being heavy or creamy.
- The red onion provides a crunchy texture and some additional flavor.
- Portion sizes should be kept modest, around 1/2 to 1 cup of the three•bean salad per serving.
- Avoid adding high•calorie or high•fat ingredients like cheese, bacon, or croutons.
- Drink water or unsweetened beverages with the salad to stay hydrated.

This three•bean salad is a nutritious, flavorful, and easy•to•digest option for those following a post•gastric bypass diet.

28. Watermelon and feta salad

Ingredient:

- 4 cups cubed seedless watermelon
- 1/2 cup crumbled low•fat feta cheese
- 2 tbsp chopped fresh mint
- 1 tbsp balsamic glaze or reduced•calorie balsamic vinaigrette
- Salt and pepper to taste

Instructions:

1. In a large bowl, gently toss together the cubed watermelon, crumbled feta cheese, and chopped fresh mint.

2. Drizzle the balsamic glaze or reduced•calorie balsamic vinaigrette over the salad.

3. Season the watermelon and feta salad with a pinch of salt and pepper.

4. Serve the salad chilled or at room temperature.

Tips for Post•Gastric Bypass:

- Watermelon is a refreshing, hydrating fruit that is low in calories and easy to digest.

- Feta cheese provides a source of protein and healthy fats that are gentle on the stomach.

- The fresh mint adds a bright, herbal flavor without the need for heavy dressings.

- The balsamic glaze or vinaigrette provides a touch of sweetness and acidity without a lot of added sugar.

- Portion sizes should be kept modest, around 1/2 to 1 cup of the salad per serving.

- Avoid pairing the salad with high•carb breads or crackers.

- Drink water or unsweetened beverages with the meal to stay hydrated.

This watermelon and feta salad is a light, refreshing, and easy•to•digest option for those following a post•gastric bypass diet.

29. Grilled vegetable skewers

Ingredient:

- 1 zucchini, cut into 1•inch pieces
- 1 yellow squash, cut into 1•inch pieces
- 1 red bell pepper, cut into 1•inch pieces
- 1 red onion, cut into 1•inch pieces
- 8 oz mushrooms, halved
- 2 tbsp olive oil
- 1 tsp dried Italian seasoning
- Salt and pepper to taste

Instructions:

1. Preheat your grill or grill pan to medium•high heat.

2. Thread the prepared vegetables onto skewers, alternating the different types.

3. In a small bowl, mix together the olive oil and dried Italian seasoning.

4. Brush the vegetable skewers with the seasoned oil, making sure to coat all sides.

5. Season the skewers with salt and pepper to taste.

6. Grill the vegetable skewers for 12•15 minutes, turning occasionally, until the vegetables are tender and lightly charred.

7. Serve the grilled vegetable skewers hot.

Tips for Post•Gastric Bypass:

- The variety of vegetables provides a range of vitamins, minerals, and fiber without a lot of calories.
- Grilling the vegetables adds a nice smoky flavor and tender texture, which can be easier to digest.
- The simple seasoning of olive oil and Italian herbs adds flavor without the need for heavy sauces or dressings.
- Portion sizes should be kept modest, around 2•3 skewers per serving.
- Avoid pairing the grilled vegetables with high•carb or high•fat accompaniments.
- Drink water or unsweetened beverages with the meal to stay hydrated.

30. Roasted vegetables (zucchini, bell peppers, onions)

Ingredient:

• 1 zucchini, cut into 1•inch pieces
• 1 red bell pepper, cut into 1•inch pieces
• 1 yellow bell pepper, cut into 1•inch pieces
• 1 red onion, cut into 1•inch pieces
• 2 tbsp olive oil
• 1 tsp dried thyme
• 1 tsp dried oregano
• Salt and pepper to taste

Instructions:

1. Preheat your oven to 400°F (200°C).

2. In a large bowl, toss the prepared zucchini, bell pepper, and onion pieces with the olive oil, dried thyme, and dried oregano. Season with salt and pepper to taste.

3. Spread the seasoned vegetables in a single layer on a large baking sheet or roasting pan.

4. Roast the vegetables for 20•25 minutes, stirring halfway, until they are tender and lightly browned. Serve the roasted vegetables hot.

Tips for Post•Gastric Bypass:

• The variety of vegetables provides a range of vitamins, minerals, and fiber without a lot of calories.

• Roasting the vegetables brings out their natural sweetness and creates a tender, easy•to•digest texture.

• The simple seasoning of olive oil, thyme, and oregano adds flavor without the need for heavy sauces or dressings.

• Portion sizes should be kept modest, around 1/2 to 1 cup of the roasted vegetables per serving.

• Avoid pairing the roasted vegetables with high•carb or high•fat accompaniments.Drink water or unsweetened beverages with the meal to stay hydrated.

31. Steamed green beans with lemon

Ingredient:

- 1 lb fresh green beans, trimmed
- 1 tbsp olive oil
- 1 tbsp fresh lemon juice
- 1 tsp grated lemon zest
- Salt and pepper to taste

Instructions:

1. Fill a medium saucepan with about 1 inch of water and bring it to a boil over high heat.

2. Add the trimmed green beans to the saucepan, cover, and steam for 5•7 minutes, or until the beans are tender•crisp.

3. Drain the steamed green beans and transfer them to a serving bowl.

4. Drizzle the olive oil and lemon juice over the green beans, and sprinkle with the grated lemon zest.

5. Toss the green beans gently to coat them with the lemon dressing.

6. Season the steamed green beans with salt and pepper to taste.

Tips for Post•Gastric Bypass:

- Green beans are a low•calorie, high•fiber vegetable that is easy to digest after surgery.
- Steaming the green beans preserves their nutrients and creates a tender, yet crisp texture.
- The lemon juice and zest add a bright, refreshing flavor without the need for heavy sauces or butter.
- Portion sizes should be kept modest, around 1/2 to 1 cup of the steamed green beans per serving.
- Avoid adding high•calorie or high•fat toppings or accompaniments.
- Drink water or unsweetened beverages with the meal to stay hydrated.

This steamed green beans with lemon dish is a simple, nutritious, and easy•to•digest side option for those following a post•gastric bypass diet.

32. Steamed asparagus with garlic

Ingredient:

- 1 lb fresh asparagus, trimmed
- 2 cloves garlic, minced
- 1 tbsp olive oil
- Salt and pepper to taste

Instructions:

1. Fill a medium saucepan with about 1 inch of water and bring to a boil.

2. Add the trimmed asparagus spears and steam for 3·5 minutes, until tender·crisp.

3. Drain the asparagus and transfer to a serving dish.

4. In a small skillet, heat the olive oil over medium heat. Add the minced garlic and cook for 1·2 minutes, until fragrant.

5. Drizzle the garlic·infused olive oil over the steamed asparagus.

6. Season with salt and pepper to taste.

Tips for post·gastric bypass:

- Asparagus is a good source of fiber, vitamins, and minerals, which can help support gut health and nutrient intake after surgery.

- The small portion size and soft texture make this a gentle, easy·to·digest option.

- The garlic adds flavor without being overpowering.

- Be sure to chew the asparagus thoroughly to aid digestion.

- Adjust seasoning to your taste preferences and tolerance level.

33. Sautéed spinach with garlic

Ingredient:

• 1 lb fresh spinach, washed and stems removed
• 2 cloves garlic, minced
• 1 tbsp olive oil
• Salt and pepper to taste

Instructions:

1. In a large skillet or sauté pan, heat the olive oil over medium heat.

2. Add the minced garlic and cook for 1•2 minutes, until fragrant.

3. Add the fresh spinach to the pan and sauté, stirring frequently, until the spinach is wilted and tender, about 3•5 minutes.

4. Season with salt and pepper to taste.

Tips for post•gastric bypass:

• Spinach is an excellent source of vitamins, minerals, and fiber, which can help support overall nutrition after surgery.

• The soft, cooked texture makes it easy to chew and digest.

• Garlic adds flavor without being overpowering, and may also have some anti•inflammatory benefits.

• Portion size is important • aim for 1/2 to 1 cup of cooked spinach per serving.

• Be sure to chew the spinach thoroughly to aid digestion.

• You can also try adding a squeeze of lemon juice or a sprinkle of parmesan cheese for extra flavor.

34. Mashed cauliflower

Ingredient:

• 1 head of cauliflower, cut into florets
• 2 tbsp unsweetened almond milk (or low•fat milk)
• 1 tbsp butter or olive oil
• Salt and pepper to taste
• Optional: garlic powder, chives, or other herbs/spices

Instructions:

1. In a large pot, bring 1•2 inches of water to a boil. Add the cauliflower florets, cover, and steam for 8•10 minutes, until very tender.

2. Drain the cauliflower and transfer to a food processor or blender.

3. Add the almond milk (or low•fat milk), butter/olive oil, and a pinch of salt and pepper. Blend or process until smooth and creamy.

4. Taste and adjust seasoning as needed, adding more salt, pepper, garlic powder, or herbs as desired.

Tips for post•gastric bypass:

• Cauliflower is an excellent source of fiber, vitamins, and minerals, making it a nutritious option.

• The soft, mashed texture is easy to chew and digest after surgery.

• The small portion size is appropriate for the reduced stomach capacity.

• The addition of healthy fats from the butter or olive oil can help increase calorie and nutrient density.

• Be sure to chew the mashed cauliflower thoroughly to aid digestion.

• You can experiment with different flavor combinations, such as adding garlic, chives, or other herbs.

Mashed cauliflower is a versatile and nutritious side dish that can be a great support for your post•gastric bypass diet.

35. Riced cauliflower

Ingredient:

• 1 head of cauliflower, cut into florets
• 1•2 tbsp olive oil or avocado oil
• Salt and pepper to taste
• Optional seasonings: garlic powder, onion powder, herbs, etc.

Instructions:

1. Place the cauliflower florets in a food processor and pulse until the cauliflower is broken down into small, rice•like pieces. Be careful not to over•process, as you don't want it to become a puree.

2. In a large skillet or sauté pan, heat the oil over medium heat.

3. Add the riced cauliflower to the pan and sauté for 5•7 minutes, stirring frequently, until the cauliflower is tender and lightly browned.

4. Season with salt, pepper, and any other desired seasonings.

Tips for post•gastric bypass:

• Cauliflower is an excellent source of fiber, vitamins, and minerals, making it a nutritious option.

• The small, rice•like texture is easy to chew and digest after surgery.

• The portion size is appropriate for the reduced stomach capacity.

• Riced cauliflower can be used as a low•carb, high•fiber substitute for rice or other grains.

• You can experiment with different flavor combinations by adding garlic, onion, herbs, or spices.

• Be sure to chew the riced cauliflower thoroughly to aid digestion.

• You can also try baking or roasting the riced cauliflower for a different texture.

Riced cauliflower is a versatile and nutritious option that can be a great support for your post•gastric bypass diet.

36. Spaghetti squash with tomato sauce

Ingredient:

• 1 medium spaghetti squash
• 1 tbsp olive oil
• 1 jar (24 oz) of your favorite low•sugar tomato sauce
• Grated parmesan cheese (optional)
• Fresh basil or oregano (optional)
• Salt and pepper to taste

Instructions:

1. Preheat your oven to 400°F (200°C).

2. Cut the spaghetti squash in half lengthwise and scoop out the seeds.

3. Place the squash halves cut•side down on a baking sheet lined with parchment paper.

4. Bake for 30•40 minutes, or until the squash is tender and easily shreds with a fork.

5. Remove the squash from the oven and let it cool slightly.

6. Using a fork, gently shred the squash flesh into long, spaghetti•like strands.

7. In a saucepan, heat the tomato sauce over medium heat until warmed through.

8. Divide the spaghetti squash strands into portions and top with the warm tomato sauce.

9. Optionally, sprinkle with grated parmesan cheese and fresh basil or oregano. Season with salt and pepper to taste.

Tips for post•gastric bypass:
• Spaghetti squash is a low•calorie, high•fiber alternative to traditional pasta, making it a great option after gastric bypass.
• The soft, noodle•like texture is easy to chew and digest.
• The portion size is appropriate for the reduced stomach capacity.
• The tomato sauce provides additional nutrients and flavor without being too heavy.
• Be sure to chew the spaghetti squash thoroughly to aid digestion.
• You can experiment with different sauce options, such as pesto or a light cream sauce, to vary the flavors.

Spaghetti squash with tomato sauce is a nutritious and satisfying meal that can support your post•gastric bypass diet.

37. Zucchini noodles with pesto

Ingredient:

- 2 medium zucchinis, spiralized or julienned into noodle•like strips
- 1/2 cup homemade or store•bought pesto (basil, kale, or other greens•based pesto)
- 2 tbsp grated parmesan cheese (optional)
- Salt and pepper to taste

Instructions:

1. Wash and trim the ends off the zucchinis. Use a spiralizer, julienne peeler, or mandoline slicer to cut the zucchinis into long, thin noodle•like strips.

2. In a large skillet or sauté pan, heat the zucchini noodles over medium heat for 2•3 minutes, just until they start to soften slightly. Be careful not to overcook them.

3. Remove the zucchini noodles from the heat and transfer them to a serving bowl.

4. Add the pesto and toss the noodles gently to coat them evenly.

5. Optionally, sprinkle the grated parmesan cheese over the top. Season with salt and pepper to taste.

Tips for post•gastric bypass:

- Zucchini noodles are a low•calorie, low•carb alternative to traditional pasta, making them a great option after gastric bypass.

- The soft, noodle•like texture is easy to chew and digest.

- The portion size is appropriate for the reduced stomach capacity.

- Pesto provides healthy fats, vitamins, and antioxidants without being too heavy.

- Be sure to chew the zucchini noodles thoroughly to aid digestion.

- You can experiment with different pesto flavors, such as kale, spinach, or sun•dried tomato.

- Adjust the portion size as needed to accommodate your individual needs and tolerance.

Zucchini noodles with pesto is a nutritious and flavorful meal that can support your post•gastric bypass diet.

38. Baked sweet potato with cinnamon

Ingredient:

- 1 medium sweet potato, scrubbed clean
- 1 tsp ground cinnamon
- 1 tbsp unsweetened almond milk (or low•fat milk)
- Salt and pepper to taste

Instructions:

1. Preheat your oven to 400°F (200°C).

2. Pierce the sweet potato several times with a fork.

3. Bake the sweet potato directly on the oven rack for 45•60 minutes, or until it's tender when pierced with a fork.

4. Remove the sweet potato from the oven and let it cool slightly.

5. Cut the sweet potato in half lengthwise.

6. Scoop out the flesh into a small bowl, leaving a thin layer of flesh attached to the skin.

7. Add the ground cinnamon and almond milk (or low•fat milk) to the sweet potato flesh. Mash and mix until well combined.

8. Season with a pinch of salt and pepper to taste. Serve the mashed sweet potato back into the potato skins, or enjoy it as a side dish.

Tips for post•gastric bypass:
- Sweet potatoes are an excellent source of fiber, vitamins, and minerals, making them a nutritious option after gastric bypass.
- The soft, mashed texture is easy to chew and digest.
- The portion size is appropriate for the reduced stomach capacity.
- Cinnamon adds flavor without the need for added sugar or butter.
- The addition of a small amount of milk helps to increase the calorie and nutrient density.
- Be sure to chew the baked sweet potato thoroughly to aid digestion.
- You can experiment with other spices, such as nutmeg or ginger, to vary the flavor.

Baked sweet potato with cinnamon is a simple, nutritious, and satisfying side dish that can support your post•gastric bypass diet.

39. Roasted Brussels sprouts

Ingredient:

- 1 lb Brussels sprouts, trimmed and halved
- 2 tbsp olive oil
- 1 tsp garlic powder (optional)
- Salt and pepper to taste

Instructions:

1. Preheat your oven to 400°F (200°C).

2. In a large bowl, toss the trimmed and halved Brussels sprouts with the olive oil, garlic powder (if using), and a pinch of salt and pepper.

3. Spread the Brussels sprouts in a single layer on a baking sheet lined with parchment paper.

4. Roast for 20•25 minutes, tossing halfway, until the Brussels sprouts are tender and lightly browned. Remove the roasted Brussels sprouts from the oven and serve immediately.

Tips for post•gastric bypass:

- Brussels sprouts are an excellent source of fiber, vitamins, and minerals, making them a nutritious option after gastric bypass.

- The roasted texture is soft and easy to chew, while still providing some crunch.

- The portion size is appropriate for the reduced stomach capacity.

- The simple seasoning with olive oil, garlic, salt, and pepper adds flavor without being too heavy.

- Be sure to chew the roasted Brussels sprouts thoroughly to aid digestion.

- You can experiment with other seasonings, such as lemon juice, parmesan cheese, or a drizzle of balsamic glaze, to vary the flavor.

- Adjust the cooking time as needed to ensure the Brussels sprouts are tender enough for your individual needs.

Roasted Brussels sprouts are a nutritious and versatile side dish that can support your post•gastric bypass diet.

40. Grilled Portobello mushroom caps

Ingredient:

• 4 large Portobello mushroom caps, stems removed
• 2 tbsp olive oil
• 1 tbsp balsamic vinegar
• 2 cloves garlic, minced
• Salt and pepper to taste

Instructions:

1. Preheat your grill or grill pan to medium•high heat.

2. In a small bowl, whisk together the olive oil, balsamic vinegar, and minced garlic.

3. Brush the Portobello mushroom caps with the oil•vinegar mixture, making sure to coat both sides.

4. Season the mushrooms with salt and pepper to taste.

5. Grill the Portobello caps for 4•5 minutes per side, or until they are tender and lightly charred. Remove the grilled mushrooms from the heat and serve immediately.

Tips for post•gastric bypass:

• Portobello mushrooms are a low•calorie, high•fiber option that can provide a satisfying, "meaty" texture after gastric bypass.

• The grilled texture is soft and easy to chew, while still providing some firmness.

• The portion size is appropriate for the reduced stomach capacity.

• The simple seasoning with olive oil, balsamic vinegar, and garlic adds flavor without being too heavy.

• Be sure to chew the grilled Portobello caps thoroughly to aid digestion.

• You can experiment with other seasonings, such as herbs, lemon juice, or a sprinkle of parmesan cheese, to vary the flavor.

• Adjust the cooking time as needed to ensure the mushrooms are tender enough for your individual needs.

41. Stuffed bell peppers with ground turkey and rice

Ingredient:

• 4 medium bell peppers, halved and seeded
• 1 lb ground turkey
• 1 cup cooked brown rice
• 1 small onion, diced
• 2 cloves garlic, minced
• 1 tsp dried oregano
• 1 tsp dried basil
• Salt and pepper to taste
• 1/2 cup shredded low•fat mozzarella cheese (optional)

Instructions:

1. Preheat your oven to 375°F (190°C).

2. In a large skillet, cook the ground turkey over medium heat until browned and cooked through, 5•7 minutes. Drain any excess fat.

3. Add the diced onion and minced garlic to the skillet. Cook for 2•3 minutes until the onion is translucent.

4. Stir in the cooked brown rice, dried oregano, and dried basil. Season with salt and pepper to taste.

5. Arrange the bell pepper halves in a baking dish. Spoon the turkey and rice mixture evenly into the pepper halves.

6. If using, sprinkle the shredded mozzarella cheese over the top of the stuffed peppers.

7. Bake for 25•30 minutes, or until the peppers are tender and the filling is heated through.

Tips for post•gastric bypass:
• Bell peppers are a good source of fiber, vitamins, and minerals, making them a nutritious option.
• Ground turkey is a lean protein that can help support muscle mass and healing after surgery.
• The rice provides complex carbohydrates and fiber to help with digestion.
• The portion size is appropriate for the reduced stomach capacity.
• The soft, cooked texture of the stuffed peppers is easy to chew and digest.

42. Stuffed zucchini boats with chicken and quinoa

Ingredient:

• 4 medium zucchinis, halved lengthwise
• 1 lb boneless, skinless chicken breasts, diced
• 1 cup cooked quinoa
• 1 small onion, diced
• 2 cloves garlic, minced
• 1 tsp dried oregano
• 1/2 tsp dried basil
• Salt and pepper to taste
• 1/4 cup shredded low•fat mozzarella cheese (optional)

Instructions:

1. Preheat your oven to 375°F (190°C).

2. Scoop out the flesh from the zucchini halves, leaving a thin shell. Chop the scooped•out zucchini flesh.

3. In a skillet, cook the diced chicken over medium heat until no longer pink, about 5•7 minutes. Transfer to a bowl.

4. In the same skillet, sauté the diced onion and garlic until translucent, about 2•3 minutes.

5. Add the chopped zucchini flesh, cooked quinoa, dried oregano, and dried basil to the skillet. Cook for 2•3 minutes, stirring frequently.

6. Transfer the quinoa mixture to the bowl with the cooked chicken. Season with salt and pepper to taste.

7. Spoon the chicken and quinoa mixture evenly into the zucchini boats.

8. Place the stuffed zucchini boats in a baking dish. If using, sprinkle the shredded mozzarella cheese over the top.

9. Bake for 20•25 minutes, or until the zucchini is tender and the filling is heated through.

Tips for post•gastric bypass:
• Zucchini boats provide a low•calorie, high•fiber vessel for the filling.
• Chicken is a lean protein that can help support muscle mass and healing after surgery.
• Quinoa is a nutrient•dense grain that provides complex carbohydrates and fiber.

43. Chicken lettuce wraps

Ingredient:

- 1 lb boneless, skinless chicken breasts, diced
- 1 tbsp olive oil
- 1 small onion, diced
- 2 cloves garlic, minced
- 1 tbsp low•sodium soy sauce or tamari
- 1 tsp sesame oil
- 1 tsp rice vinegar
- 1 tsp grated ginger (or 1/2 tsp ground ginger)
- Salt and pepper to taste
- 8•10 large lettuce leaves (such as romaine, bibb, or butter lettuce)

Instructions:

1. In a large skillet or wok, heat the olive oil over medium•high heat.

2. Add the diced chicken and sauté until cooked through, about 5•7 minutes.

3. Add the diced onion and minced garlic to the skillet. Cook for 2•3 minutes until the onion is translucent.

4. In a small bowl, whisk together the soy sauce, sesame oil, rice vinegar, and grated ginger.

5. Pour the sauce mixture into the skillet with the chicken and onions. Stir to combine and let the flavors meld for 2•3 minutes.

6. Season the chicken mixture with salt and pepper to taste. To serve, spoon the chicken mixture into the lettuce leaves and enjoy.

Tips for post•gastric bypass:

- Lettuce leaves provide a low•calorie, high•fiber "wrap" for the chicken filling.

- Chicken is a lean protein that can help support muscle mass and healing after surgery.

- The small portion size is appropriate for the reduced stomach capacity.

- The soft, cooked texture of the chicken is easy to chew and digest.

- Be sure to chew the lettuce wraps thoroughly to aid digestion.

44. Turkey roll•ups with cheese and vegetables

Ingredient:

• 8 slices of deli turkey (about 4 oz)
• 2 oz low•fat cheddar or Swiss cheese, sliced
• 1/2 cup diced cucumber
• 1/4 cup diced bell pepper
• 1 tbsp chopped fresh parsley (optional)
• Salt and pepper to taste

Instructions:
1. Lay the turkey slices flat on a clean surface.

2. Place a slice of cheese on each turkey slice.

3. Divide the diced cucumber and bell pepper evenly among the turkey slices, placing them in a line near the center of the slice.

4. Sprinkle the chopped parsley (if using) over the vegetables.

5. Carefully roll up each turkey slice, starting from the short end and rolling tightly to enclose the filling. Secure the roll•ups with toothpicks, if needed.

Tips for post•gastric bypass:
• Turkey is a lean protein that can help support muscle mass and healing after surgery.

• The cheese provides healthy fats and additional protein.

• The vegetables add fiber, vitamins, and minerals without being too bulky.

• The small, bite•sized roll•ups are easy to chew and digest.

• The portion size is appropriate for the reduced stomach capacity.

• Be sure to chew the roll•ups thoroughly to aid digestion.

• You can experiment with different vegetable combinations, such as shredded carrots, diced tomatoes, or sliced avocado.

• Avoid any crunchy or raw vegetables that may be difficult to digest in the early stages of recovery.

Turkey roll•ups with cheese and vegetables can be a nutritious and satisfying snack or light meal to support your post•gastric bypass diet.

45. Shrimp stir•fry with vegetables

Ingredient:

- 1 lb peeled and deveined shrimp
- 2 tbsp low•sodium soy sauce or tamari
- 1 tsp sesame oil
- 1 tbsp olive oil
- 2 cloves garlic, minced
- 1 inch piece of ginger, peeled and grated
- 1 cup sliced mushrooms
- 1 cup broccoli florets
- 1 cup sliced bell peppers
- 1/2 cup snow peas or snap peas
- 2 tbsp low•sodium chicken or vegetable broth
- Salt and pepper to taste
- Chopped green onions or cilantro for garnish (optional)

Instructions:

1. In a small bowl, combine the shrimp, soy sauce, and sesame oil. Set aside.

2. Heat the olive oil in a large skillet or wok over high heat.

3. Add the minced garlic and grated ginger to the pan and cook for 30 seconds, stirring constantly.

4. Add the shrimp mixture to the pan and cook for 2•3 minutes, until the shrimp start to turn pink.

5. Add the sliced mushrooms, broccoli, bell peppers, and snow peas to the pan. Stir•fry for 3•5 minutes, until the vegetables are tender•crisp.

6. Pour in the chicken or vegetable broth and stir to combine. Cook for an additional 1•2 minutes, until the sauce has thickened slightly.

7. Season with salt and pepper to taste.

8. Serve the shrimp stir•fry immediately, garnished with chopped green onions or cilantro, if desired.

Tips for post•gastric bypass:

- Shrimp is a lean protein that can help support muscle mass and healing after surgery.
- The variety of vegetables provides fiber, vitamins, and minerals without being too bulky.

46. Tofu stir•fry with vegetables

Ingredient:

- 1 block (14 oz) firm or extra•firm tofu, diced
- 2 tbsp low•sodium soy sauce or tamari
- 1 tsp sesame oil
- 1 tbsp olive oil
- 2 cloves garlic, minced
- 1 inch piece of ginger, peeled and grated
- 1 cup sliced mushrooms
- 1 cup broccoli florets
- 1 cup sliced bell peppers
- 1/2 cup snow peas or snap peas
- 2 tbsp low•sodium vegetable broth
- Salt and pepper to taste
- Chopped green onions or cilantro for garnish (optional)

Instructions:

1. In a small bowl, combine the diced tofu, soy sauce, and sesame oil. Set aside.

2. Heat the olive oil in a large skillet or wok over high heat.

3. Add the minced garlic and grated ginger to the pan and cook for 30 seconds, stirring constantly.

4. Add the tofu mixture to the pan and cook for 2•3 minutes, until the tofu starts to brown.

5. Add the sliced mushrooms, broccoli, bell peppers, and snow peas to the pan. Stir•fry for 3•5 minutes, until the vegetables are tender•crisp.

6. Pour in the vegetable broth and stir to combine. Cook for an additional 1•2 minutes, until the sauce has thickened slightly.

7. Season with salt and pepper to taste.

8. Serve the tofu stir•fry immediately, garnished with chopped green onions or cilantro, if desired.

Tofu stir•fry with vegetables is a nutritious and flavorful vegetarian option that can support your post•gastric bypass diet.

47. Beef and broccoli stir•fry

Ingredient:

• 1 lb flank steak or sirloin, thinly sliced
• 2 tbsp low•sodium soy sauce or tamari
• 1 tsp sesame oil
• 1 tbsp olive oil
• 2 cloves garlic, minced
• 1 inch piece of ginger, peeled and grated
• 1 cup broccoli florets
• 1 cup sliced mushrooms
• 1/2 cup sliced bell peppers
• 2 tbsp low•sodium beef or chicken broth
• Salt and pepper to taste
• Chopped green onions for garnish (optional)

Instructions:

1. In a small bowl, combine the sliced beef, soy sauce, and sesame oil. Set aside.

2. Heat the olive oil in a large skillet or wok over high heat.

3. Add the minced garlic and grated ginger to the pan and cook for 30 seconds, stirring constantly.

4. Add the marinated beef to the pan and cook for 2•3 minutes, until the beef is browned and cooked through.

5. Add the broccoli florets, sliced mushrooms, and bell peppers to the pan. Stir•fry for 3•5 minutes, until the vegetables are tender•crisp.

6. Pour in the beef or chicken broth and stir to

combine. Cook for an additional 1•2 minutes, until the sauce has thickened slightly.
7. Season with salt and pepper to taste.

8. Serve the beef and broccoli stir•fry immediately, garnished with chopped green onions, if desired.

Beef and broccoli stir•fry is a nutritious and flavorful option that can support your post•gastric bypass diet.

48. Grilled salmon with dill and lemon

Ingredient:

- 4 (4 oz) salmon fillets
- 2 tbsp olive oil
- 2 tbsp fresh dill, chopped
- 1 tbsp lemon juice
- 1 tsp lemon zest
- Salt and pepper to taste

Instructions:
1. Preheat your grill or grill pan to medium•high heat.

2. In a small bowl, mix together the olive oil, chopped dill, lemon juice, and lemon zest.

3. Season the salmon fillets with salt and pepper.

4. Grill the salmon for 4•6 minutes per side, or until it flakes easily with a fork.

5. Brush the salmon with the dill•lemon mixture during the last 2 minutes of cooking.

6. Serve the grilled salmon immediately, with any remaining dill•lemon sauce drizzled over the top.

Tips for post•gastric bypass:
- Salmon is an excellent source of lean protein, healthy fats, and essential vitamins and minerals, making it a great choice after gastric bypass.

- The grilled texture is soft and easy to chew, while still providing some firmness.

- The portion size is appropriate for the reduced stomach capacity.

- The simple seasoning with dill and lemon adds flavor without being too heavy.

- Be sure to chew the grilled salmon thoroughly to aid digestion.

- You can experiment with other herbs, such as parsley or basil, to vary the flavor.

- Avoid any heavy sauces or toppings that may be difficult to digest in the early stages of recovery.

49. Baked cod with breadcrumbs and herbs

Ingredient:

- 4 (4 oz) cod fillets
- 1/4 cup panko breadcrumbs
- 2 tbsp grated parmesan cheese
- 1 tbsp chopped fresh parsley
- 1 tbsp chopped fresh dill
- 1 tbsp olive oil
- 1 tbsp lemon juice
- Salt and pepper to taste

Instructions:

1. Preheat your oven to 400°F (200°C).

2. In a shallow bowl, mix together the panko breadcrumbs, parmesan cheese, chopped parsley, and chopped dill.

3. Drizzle the olive oil and lemon juice over the cod fillets and season with salt and pepper.

4. Gently press the breadcrumb mixture onto the top of the cod fillets, covering them completely.

5. Place the breaded cod fillets on a baking sheet lined with parchment paper.

6. Bake for 12•15 minutes, or until the cod is cooked through and the breadcrumbs are golden brown. Serve the baked cod immediately.

Tips for post•gastric bypass:
- Cod is a lean, flaky white fish that is easy to chew and digest after gastric bypass surgery.
- The breadcrumb and herb topping adds flavor and texture without being too heavy.
- The portion size is appropriate for the reduced stomach capacity.
- Be sure to chew the baked cod thoroughly to aid digestion.
- Avoid any heavy or creamy sauces that may be difficult to digest in the early stages of recovery.
- You can experiment with different herb combinations, such as basil and oregano, to vary the flavor.
- If the breadcrumbs are too crunchy, you can try pulsing them in a food processor to create a finer texture.

50. Tilapia fish tacos with cabbage slaw

Ingredient:

- 1 lb tilapia fillets, cut into 1·inch pieces
- 1 tbsp olive oil
- 1 tsp chili powder
- 1/2 tsp cumin
- Salt and pepper to taste
- 8 small corn tortillas or lettuce leaves
- For the Cabbage Slaw:
- 2 cups shredded green cabbage
- 1/4 cup shredded carrots
- 2 tbsp plain Greek yogurt
- 1 tbsp lime juice
- 1 tbsp chopped cilantro
- Salt and pepper to taste

Instructions:

1. In a medium bowl, toss the tilapia pieces with the olive oil, chili powder, cumin, salt, and pepper.

2. Heat a large skillet over medium·high heat. Add the seasoned tilapia and cook for 3·4 minutes per side, until the fish flakes easily with a fork.

3. In a separate bowl, mix together the shredded cabbage, carrots, Greek yogurt, lime juice, and chopped cilantro. Season with salt and pepper.

4. To assemble the tacos, place a portion of the tilapia in the center of each corn tortilla or lettuce leaf. Top with a spoonful of the cabbage slaw. Serve the fish tacos immediately.

Tips for post·gastric bypass:

- Tilapia is a lean, mild·flavored fish that is easy to chew and digest after gastric bypass surgery.

- The cabbage slaw provides a crunchy, refreshing contrast to the soft fish, without being too bulky.

- The small corn tortillas or lettuce leaves are a low·calorie, low·carb option for the "taco" shell.

- The portion size is appropriate for the reduced stomach capacity. Be sure to chew the fish tacos thoroughly to aid digestion.

51. Tuna patties

Ingredient:

- 2 (5 oz) cans of tuna, drained and flaked
- 1 egg, lightly beaten
- 2 tbsp whole wheat breadcrumbs
- 2 tbsp finely chopped onion
- 1 tbsp chopped fresh parsley
- 1 tsp Dijon mustard
- Salt and pepper to taste
- 1 tbsp olive oil

Instructions:

1. In a medium bowl, combine the flaked tuna, beaten egg, breadcrumbs, chopped onion, parsley, and Dijon mustard. Season with salt and pepper.

2. Gently mix the ingredients together until well combined, being careful not to overmix.

3. Form the mixture into 4 equal-sized patties, about 1/2 inch thick.

4. In a non-stick skillet, heat the olive oil over medium heat.

5. Carefully add the tuna patties to the hot oil and cook for 3-4 minutes per side, or until golden brown and heated through. Serve the tuna patties immediately.

Tips for post-gastric bypass:

- Tuna is a lean protein that can help support muscle mass and healing after gastric bypass surgery.

- The small, patty-like size is easy to chew and digest.

- The portion size is appropriate for the reduced stomach capacity.

- The breadcrumbs provide a light, crispy texture without being too heavy.

- Be sure to chew the tuna patties thoroughly to aid digestion.

- You can experiment with different herbs and spices, such as dill, lemon zest, or garlic powder, to vary the flavor.

- Avoid any heavy or creamy sauces that may be difficult to digest in the early stages of recovery.

52. Salmon patties

Ingredient:

• 2 (5 oz) cans of salmon, drained and flaked
• 1 egg, lightly beaten
• 2 tbsp whole wheat breadcrumbs
• 2 tbsp finely chopped onion
• 1 tbsp chopped fresh dill (or 1 tsp dried dill)
• 1 tsp Dijon mustard
• Salt and pepper to taste
• 1 tbsp olive oil

Instructions:

1. In a medium bowl, combine the flaked salmon, beaten egg, breadcrumbs, chopped onion, dill, and Dijon mustard. Season with salt and pepper.

2. Gently mix the ingredients together until well combined, being careful not to overmix.

3. Form the mixture into 4 equal•sized patties, about 1/2 inch thick.

4. In a non•stick skillet, heat the olive oil over medium heat.

5. Carefully add the salmon patties to the hot oil and cook for 3•4 minutes per side, or until golden brown and heated through. Serve the salmon patties immediately.

Tips for post•gastric bypass:

• Salmon is an excellent source of lean protein, healthy fats, and essential vitamins and minerals, making it a great choice after gastric bypass.

• The small, patty•like size is easy to chew and digest.

• The portion size is appropriate for the reduced stomach capacity.

• The breadcrumbs provide a light, crispy texture without being too heavy.

• The dill adds flavor without being overpowering.

• Be sure to chew the salmon patties thoroughly to aid digestion.

• You can experiment with other herbs and spices, such as lemon zest or garlic powder, to vary the flavor.

53. Turkey burger with lettuce wrap

Ingredient:

- 1 lb ground turkey
- 1 tbsp Dijon mustard
- 1 tsp dried oregano
- 1/2 tsp garlic powder
- Salt and pepper to taste
- 8•10 large lettuce leaves (such as romaine, bibb, or butter lettuce)
- Optional toppings: sliced tomato, onion, pickles, etc.

Instructions:

1. In a medium bowl, combine the ground turkey, Dijon mustard, dried oregano, garlic powder, and a pinch of salt and pepper. Mix gently until just combined, being careful not to overmix.

2. Divide the turkey mixture into 4 equal•sized patties, about 1/2 inch thick.

3. Heat a non•stick skillet or grill pan over medium•high heat.

4. Cook the turkey patties for 4•5 minutes per side, or until they are cooked through and no longer pink in the center.

5. Place each cooked turkey burger on a large lettuce leaf.

6. Top the turkey burgers with your desired toppings, such as sliced tomato, onion, or pickles. Wrap the lettuce around the burger and enjoy.

Tips for post•gastric bypass:

- Ground turkey is a lean protein that can help support muscle mass and healing after gastric bypass surgery.

- The small, burger•sized portion is appropriate for the reduced stomach capacity.

- The lettuce wrap provides a low•calorie, low•carb alternative to a traditional bun.

- The soft, cooked texture of the turkey burger is easy to chew and digest.

- Be sure to chew the turkey burgers thoroughly to aid digestion.

- Avoid any heavy or creamy toppings that may be difficult to digest in the early stages of recovery.

54. Veggie burger with lettuce wrap

Ingredient:

• 1 (15 oz) can black beans, drained and rinsed
• 1 cup cooked quinoa
• 1/2 cup rolled oats
• 1/4 cup finely chopped onion
• 2 cloves garlic, minced
• 1 tsp ground cumin
• 1/2 tsp chili powder
• Salt and pepper to taste
• 8•10 large lettuce leaves (such as romaine, bibb, or butter lettuce)
• Optional toppings: sliced tomato, avocado, pickles, etc.

Instructions:

1. In a medium bowl, mash the black beans with a fork or potato masher until slightly chunky.

2. Add the cooked quinoa, rolled oats, chopped onion, minced garlic, cumin, chili powder, and a pinch of salt and pepper. Mix well until the ingredients are fully combined.

3. Divide the veggie burger mixture into 4 equal•sized patties, about 1/2 inch thick.

4. Heat a non•stick skillet or grill pan over medium•high heat.

5. Cook the veggie patties for 4•5 minutes per side, or until they are heated through and lightly browned.

6. Place each cooked veggie burger on a large lettuce leaf.

7. Top the veggie burgers with your desired toppings, such as sliced tomato or avocado.

8. Wrap the lettuce around the burger and enjoy.

Tips for post•gastric bypass:

• Black beans and quinoa provide plant•based protein and fiber to support overall nutrition after gastric bypass.

• The small, burger•sized portion is appropriate for the reduced stomach capacity.

• The lettuce wrap provides a low•calorie, low•carb alternative to a traditional bun.

55. Black bean burger with avocado

Ingredient:

- 1 (15 oz) can black beans, drained and rinsed
- 1/2 cup cooked quinoa
- 1/4 cup rolled oats
- 1 egg, lightly beaten
- 2 tbsp finely chopped onion
- 2 cloves garlic, minced
- 1 tsp ground cumin
- 1/2 tsp chili powder
- Salt and pepper to taste
- 1 avocado, sliced
- 4 large lettuce leaves (such as romaine or bibb)

Instructions:

1. In a medium bowl, mash the black beans with a fork or potato masher until slightly chunky.

2. Add the cooked quinoa, rolled oats, beaten egg, chopped onion, minced garlic, cumin, chili powder, and a pinch of salt and pepper. Mix well until the ingredients are fully combined.

3. Divide the black bean mixture into 4 equal•sized patties, about 1/2 inch thick.

4. Heat a non•stick skillet or grill pan over medium•high heat.

5. Cook the black bean patties for 4•5 minutes per side, or until they are heated through and lightly browned.

6. Place each cooked black bean burger on a large lettuce leaf.

7. Top the burgers with sliced avocado. Wrap the lettuce around the burger and enjoy.

Tips for post•gastric bypass:

- Black beans provide plant•based protein and fiber to support overall nutrition after gastric bypass.

- The quinoa and oats help bind the patties together without the need for a lot of breadcrumbs or fillers.

- The small, burger•sized portion is appropriate for the reduced stomach capacity.

56. Chicken fajitas with bell peppers and onions

Ingredient:

• 1 lb boneless, skinless chicken breasts, sliced into thin strips
• 2 tbsp olive oil
• 1 tbsp lime juice
• 1 tsp chili powder
• 1 tsp ground cumin
• 1/2 tsp garlic powder
• Salt and pepper to taste
• 1 red bell pepper, sliced
• 1 green bell pepper, sliced
• 1 onion, sliced
• 8•10 large lettuce leaves (such as romaine or bibb)
• Optional toppings: diced avocado, salsa, plain Greek yogurt

Instructions:

1. In a large bowl, combine the sliced chicken, olive oil, lime juice, chili powder, cumin, garlic powder, and a pinch of salt and pepper. Toss to coat the chicken.

2. Heat a large skillet or grill pan over medium•high heat.

3. Add the seasoned chicken to the hot pan and cook for 5•7 minutes, stirring occasionally, until the chicken is cooked through.

4. Remove the chicken from the pan and set aside.

5. In the same pan, sauté the sliced bell peppers and onion for 3•5 minutes, until they are tender•crisp.

6. Return the cooked chicken to the pan with the vegetables and toss to combine.

7. To serve, place a portion of the chicken and vegetable mixture into a large lettuce leaf.

8. Top the fajitas with your desired toppings, such as diced avocado, salsa, or plain Greek yogurt.

Chicken fajitas with bell peppers and onions can be a nutritious and satisfying option to support your post•gastric bypass diet.

57. Steak fajitas with bell peppers and onions

Ingredient:

- 1 lb lean flank steak, thinly sliced
- 2 bell peppers, thinly sliced
- 1 onion, thinly sliced
- 2 tbsp olive oil
- 1 tsp cumin
- 1 tsp chili powder
- 1/2 tsp garlic powder
- Salt and pepper to taste
- 4•6 small low•carb tortillas or lettuce wraps

Instructions:

1. In a large skillet or wok, heat the olive oil over medium•high heat.

2. Add the sliced steak, bell peppers, and onions. Season with the cumin, chili powder, garlic powder, salt, and pepper.

3. Sauté the mixture, stirring frequently, until the steak is cooked through and the vegetables are tender, about 8•10 minutes.

4. Serve the steak and vegetable mixture in the small low•carb tortillas or lettuce wraps.

Tips:
• Use lean flank steak to keep the fat and calories low.

• Slice the vegetables and steak thinly so they cook quickly.

• Stick to small portions of the tortillas or use lettuce wraps to keep carbs in check.

• Pair with a side salad or roasted veggies for a complete post•op friendly meal.

58. Shrimp fajitas with bell peppers and onions

Ingredient:

- 1 lb peeled and deveined shrimp
- 2 bell peppers, thinly sliced
- 1 onion, thinly sliced
- 2 tbsp olive oil
- 1 tsp cumin
- 1 tsp chili powder
- 1/2 tsp garlic powder
- Salt and pepper to taste
- 4•6 small low•carb tortillas or lettuce wraps

Instructions:

1. In a large skillet or wok, heat the olive oil over medium•high heat.

2. Add the shrimp, bell peppers, and onions. Season with the cumin, chili powder, garlic powder, salt, and pepper.

3. Sauté the mixture, stirring frequently, until the shrimp are cooked through and the vegetables are tender, about 6•8 minutes.

4. Serve the shrimp and vegetable mixture in the small low•carb tortillas or lettuce wraps.

Tips:
• Use peeled and deveined shrimp to make it easier to digest.

• Slice the vegetables thinly so they cook quickly.

• Stick to small portions of the tortillas or use lettuce wraps to keep carbs in check.

• Pair with a side salad or roasted veggies for a complete post•op friendly meal.

59. Chicken enchiladas with salsa verde

Ingredient:

- 2 cups shredded cooked chicken breast
- 1 cup salsa verde (green salsa)
- 1/2 cup low•fat sour cream
- 1/4 cup shredded low•fat cheddar cheese
- 4•6 small low•carb tortillas or lettuce leaves

For the Salsa Verde:
- 1 lb tomatillos, husks removed and rinsed
- 1 jalapeño, seeded and diced
- 1/2 onion, diced
- 2 cloves garlic, minced
- 1/4 cup chopped cilantro
- Juice of 1 lime
- Salt and pepper to taste

Instructions:

1. Preheat oven to 375°F.

2. Make the salsa verde: In a blender or food processor, combine the tomatillos, jalapeño, onion, garlic, cilantro, and lime juice. Blend until smooth. Season with salt and pepper.

3. In a bowl, mix the shredded chicken with 1/2 cup of the salsa verde and the sour cream.

4. Spoon the chicken mixture into the low•carb tortillas or lettuce leaves. Roll up and place seam•side down in a baking dish.

5. Pour the remaining salsa verde over the enchiladas and top with the shredded cheese.

6. Bake for 15•20 minutes, until heated through and the cheese is melted.

Tips:
- Use low•carb tortillas or lettuce leaves to keep the carbs down.
- Stick to small portions to avoid overeating.
- Pair with a side salad or roasted vegetables for a complete post•op friendly meal.

60. Beef enchiladas with red sauce

Ingredient:

- 1 lb lean ground beef
- 1 onion, diced
- 2 cloves garlic, minced
- 1 tbsp chili powder
- 1 tsp cumin
- Salt and pepper to taste
- 1 cup low•fat shredded cheddar cheese
- 4•6 small low•carb tortillas or lettuce leaves
- 1 (15 oz) can red enchilada sauce

For the Red Sauce:

- 1 (15 oz) can tomato sauce
- 1 tbsp chili powder
- 1 tsp cumin
- 1 tsp garlic powder
- Salt and pepper to taste

Instructions:

1. Preheat oven to 375°F.

2. In a skillet over medium heat, cook the ground beef, onion, and garlic until the beef is browned and the onions are translucent, about 5•7 minutes. Drain any excess fat.

3. Season the beef mixture with the chili powder, cumin, salt, and pepper.

4. Make the red sauce: In a small bowl, whisk together the tomato sauce, chili powder, cumin, garlic powder, salt, and pepper.

5. Spoon the beef mixture into the low•carb tortillas or lettuce leaves. Roll up and place seam•side down in a baking dish.

6. Pour the red enchilada sauce over the enchiladas and top with the shredded cheese.

7. Bake for 15•20 minutes, until heated through and the cheese is melted.

Tips:
- Use lean ground beef to keep the fat and calories low.
- Stick to small portions of the tortillas or use lettuce leaves to keep carbs in check.
- Pair with a side salad or roasted vegetables for a complete post•op friendly meal.

61. Cheese quesadillas

Ingredient:

- 4•6 small low•carb tortillas
- 1 cup shredded low•fat cheddar or Monterey Jack cheese
- 2 tbsp low•fat sour cream (optional)
- Salsa or guacamole for serving (optional)

Instructions:

1. Preheat a non•stick skillet or griddle over medium heat.

2. Place one low•carb tortilla in the skillet. Sprinkle 2•3 tablespoons of the shredded cheese evenly over half of the tortilla.

3. Fold the other half of the tortilla over the cheese•topped half to create a half•moon shape.

4. Cook the quesadilla for 2•3 minutes per side, or until the tortilla is lightly browned and the cheese is melted.

5. Remove the quesadilla from the skillet and cut it in half.

6. Repeat the process with the remaining tortillas and cheese.

7. Serve the quesadilla halves warm, with a dollop of low•fat sour cream, salsa, or guacamole on the side, if desired.

Tips:

- Use small, low•carb tortillas to keep the portion size and carb content in check.

- Opt for low•fat or reduced•fat cheese to keep the fat and calories lower.

- Stick to 1•2 quesadilla halves per serving to avoid overeating.

- Pair the quesadillas with a side salad or roasted vegetables for a more complete post•op friendly meal.

62. Chicken quesadillas

Ingredient:

- 4•6 small low•carb tortillas
- 1 cup shredded cooked chicken breast
- 1/2 cup shredded low•fat cheddar or Monterey Jack cheese
- 2 tbsp low•fat sour cream (optional)
- Salsa or guacamole for serving (optional)

Instructions:

1. Preheat a non•stick skillet or griddle over medium heat.

2. Place one low•carb tortilla in the skillet. Sprinkle 2•3 tablespoons of the shredded chicken and 1•2 tablespoons of the shredded cheese evenly over half of the tortilla.

3. Fold the other half of the tortilla over the chicken and cheese•topped half to create a half•moon shape.

4. Cook the quesadilla for 2•3 minutes per side, or until the tortilla is lightly browned and the cheese is melted.

5. Remove the quesadilla from the skillet and cut it in half.

6. Repeat the process with the remaining tortillas, chicken, and cheese.

7. Serve the quesadilla halves warm, with a dollop of low•fat sour cream, salsa, or guacamole on the side, if desired.

Tips:

• Use small, low•carb tortillas to keep the portion size and carb content in check.

• Opt for shredded cooked chicken breast to keep the protein high and the fat low.

• Use low•fat or reduced•fat cheese to keep the fat and calories lower.

• Stick to 1•2 quesadilla halves per serving to avoid overeating.

• Pair the quesadillas with a side salad or roasted vegetables for a more complete post•op friendly meal.

63. Bean and cheese burritos

Ingredient:

- 4•6 small low•carb tortillas
- 1 (15 oz) can low•sodium black beans, rinsed and drained
- 1/2 cup shredded low•fat cheddar or Monterey Jack cheese
- 2 tbsp low•fat sour cream (optional)
- Salsa or guacamole for serving (optional)

Instructions:

1. In a medium bowl, mash the black beans with a fork or potato masher until they are slightly chunky.

2. Place one low•carb tortilla on a flat surface. Spoon 2•3 tablespoons of the mashed black beans onto the center of the tortilla.

3. Sprinkle 1•2 tablespoons of the shredded cheese over the beans.

4. Fold the bottom of the tortilla up over the filling, then fold in the sides and continue rolling up tightly to create a burrito.

5. Repeat the process with the remaining tortillas, beans, and cheese.

6. Serve the burritos warm, with a dollop of low•fat sour cream, salsa, or guacamole on the side, if desired.

Tips:

- Use small, low•carb tortillas to keep the portion size and carb content in check.

- Opt for low•sodium black beans to reduce the sodium intake.

- Use low•fat or reduced•fat cheese to keep the fat and calories lower.

- Stick to 1•2 burritos per serving to avoid overeating.

- Pair the burritos with a side salad or roasted vegetables for a more complete post•op friendly meal.

64. Chicken burritos with rice and beans

Ingredient:

- 4·6 small low·carb tortillas
- 1 cup cooked shredded chicken breast
- 1/2 cup cooked low·carb cauliflower rice (or brown rice)
- 1/2 cup low·sodium black beans, rinsed and drained
- 1/4 cup shredded low·fat cheddar or Monterey Jack cheese
- 2 tbsp low·fat sour cream (optional)
- Salsa or guacamole for serving (optional)

Instructions:

1. In a medium bowl, mix together the shredded chicken, cauliflower rice (or brown rice), and black beans.

2. Place one low·carb tortilla on a flat surface. Spoon 2·3 tablespoons of the chicken, rice, and bean mixture onto the center of the tortilla.

3. Sprinkle 1·2 tablespoons of the shredded cheese over the filling.

4. Fold the bottom of the tortilla up over the filling, then fold in the sides and continue rolling up tightly to create a burrito.

5. Repeat the process with the remaining tortillas, filling, and cheese.

6. Serve the burritos warm, with a dollop of low·fat sour cream, salsa, or guacamole on the side, if desired.

Tips:

- Use small, low·carb tortillas to keep the portion size and carb content in check.

- Opt for cooked shredded chicken breast to keep the protein high and the fat low.

- Use low·carb cauliflower rice or brown rice to provide fiber and nutrients.

- Choose low·sodium black beans to reduce the sodium intake.

- Use low·fat or reduced·fat cheese to keep the fat and calories lower.

- Stick to 1·2 burritos per serving to avoid overeating.

- Pair the burritos with a side salad or roasted vegetables for a more complete post·op friendly meal.

65. Taco salad with ground turkey, lettuce, and salsa

Ingredient:

- 4 cups chopped romaine or mixed greens
- 1 lb lean ground turkey
- 1 tsp chili powder
- 1/2 tsp cumin
- 1/4 tsp garlic powder
- Salt and pepper to taste
- 1/2 cup diced tomatoes or salsa
- 2 tbsp shredded low•fat cheddar or Monterey Jack cheese
- 2 tbsp low•fat sour cream (optional)

Instructions:

1. In a skillet over medium•high heat, cook the ground turkey, breaking it up as it cooks, until it's browned and cooked through, about 5•7 minutes.

2. Drain any excess fat from the skillet, then season the turkey with the chili powder, cumin, garlic powder, salt, and pepper.

3. Divide the chopped romaine or mixed greens between 4 bowls.

4. Top each salad with 1/4 of the seasoned ground turkey.

5. Drizzle 2 tablespoons of salsa or diced tomatoes over the top of each salad.

6. Sprinkle 1/2 tablespoon of the shredded cheese over each salad.

7. If desired, top each salad with 1 tablespoon of low•fat sour cream.

Tips:

- Use lean ground turkey to keep the fat and calories low.
- Stick to a 4•cup portion of greens to avoid overeating.
- Opt for a low•carb salsa or diced tomatoes to keep the carbs in check.
- Use a small amount of low•fat cheese and sour cream to add flavor without too many extra calories.
- This salad can be a complete meal on its own, or you can serve it with a small portion of roasted vegetables for a more filling post•op friendly meal.

66. Ceviche with shrimp or fish

Ingredient:

• 1 lb peeled and deveined shrimp or white fish (such as tilapia or halibut), cut into 1·inch pieces
• 1 cup fresh lime juice (about 6·8 limes)
• 1/2 cup diced red onion
• 1 jalapeño, seeded and diced (optional)
• 1 cup diced tomatoes
• 1/4 cup chopped cilantro
• Salt and pepper to taste
• Lettuce leaves or endive leaves for serving

Instructions:

1. In a large non·reactive bowl (glass or stainless steel), combine the shrimp or fish, lime juice, red onion, and jalapeño (if using). Cover and refrigerate for 30·60 minutes, or until the seafood is opaque and "cooked" through the acid in the lime juice.

2. Drain any excess lime juice from the bowl. Add the diced tomatoes and chopped cilantro. Season with salt and pepper to taste.

3. Serve the ceviche in lettuce or endive leaves, or on its own as a salad.

Tips:

• Use peeled and deveined shrimp or white fish to make it easier to digest.

• Stick to a 4·6 oz portion of the ceviche to avoid overeating.

• The acid in the lime juice "cooks" the seafood, so there's no need for additional cooking.

• Omit the jalapeño if you prefer a milder flavor.

• Serve the ceviche in lettuce or endive leaves to keep the carbs low.

• Pair the ceviche with a side salad or roasted vegetables for a more complete post·op friendly meal.

67. Gazpacho (cold vegetable soup)

Ingredient:

- 2 lbs ripe tomatoes, diced
- 1 cucumber, peeled, seeded, and diced
- 1 red bell pepper, diced
- 1 small red onion, diced
- 2 cloves garlic, minced
- 2 tbsp red wine vinegar
- 2 tbsp olive oil
- 1 tsp Dijon mustard
- 1/4 cup chopped fresh basil or cilantro
- Salt and pepper to taste
- Lime wedges for serving (optional)

Instructions:

1. In a large bowl, combine the diced tomatoes, cucumber, bell pepper, onion, and garlic.

2. In a small bowl, whisk together the red wine vinegar, olive oil, and Dijon mustard. Pour the dressing over the vegetable mixture and stir to coat.

3. Stir in the chopped basil or cilantro and season with salt and pepper t
o taste.

4. Cover the gazpacho and refrigerate for at least 2 hours, or up to 24 hours, to allow the flavors to meld.

5. Serve the gazpacho chilled, with lime wedges on the side if desired.

Tips:

- Use ripe, in•season tomatoes for the best flavor.
- Peel and seed the cucumber to make it easier to digest.
- Stick to a 1•cup portion of the gazpacho to avoid overeating.
- The gazpacho can be a light and refreshing starter or a main course when paired with a protein•rich side, such as grilled shrimp or chicken.
- Garnish with a sprinkle of fresh herbs or a dollop of low•fat Greek yogurt for added flavor and nutrition.

68. Stuffed grape leaves (dolmas)

Ingredient:

- 1 (16 oz) jar of grape leaves, drained and rinsed
- 1/2 lb ground turkey or lean ground beef
- 1/2 cup cooked cauliflower rice (or brown rice)
- 1/4 cup diced onion
- 2 cloves garlic, minced
- 2 tbsp chopped fresh parsley
- 1 tsp lemon juice
- 1/4 tsp ground cinnamon
- Salt and pepper to taste
- Lemon wedges for serving (optional)

Instructions:

1. In a medium bowl, combine the ground turkey or beef, cauliflower rice (or brown rice), onion, garlic, parsley, lemon juice, cinnamon, salt, and pepper. Mix well.

2. Lay a grape leaf shiny•side down on a flat surface. Place about 1•2 tablespoons of the filling near the stem end of the leaf. Fold the stem end over the filling, then fold in the sides and roll up tightly to enclose the filling.

3. Repeat with the remaining grape leaves and filling.

4. Arrange the stuffed grape leaves seam•side down in a single layer in a saucepan or baking dish.

5. Cover the grape leaves with water or broth and bring to a simmer over medium heat. Reduce heat to low, cover, and simmer for 30•40 minutes, or until the grape leaves are tender.

6. Carefully remove the grape leaves from the liquid and serve warm, with lemon wedges on the side if desired.

Tips:

- Use ground turkey or lean ground beef to keep the fat and calories low.
- Opt for cauliflower rice or brown rice to provide fiber and nutrients.
- Stick to 2•3 grape leaves per serving to avoid overeating.
- Serve the grape leaves as a side dish or a light main course, paired with a salad or roasted vegetables.

69. Baked falafel with tzatziki sauce

Ingredient:

For the Falafel:
• 1 (15 oz) can chickpeas, rinsed and drained
• 1/2 cup cooked cauliflower rice (or brown rice)
• 2 tbsp chopped fresh parsley
• 1 tbsp lemon juice
• 1 tsp ground cumin
• 1/2 tsp garlic powder
• 1/4 tsp cayenne pepper (optional)
• Salt and pepper to taste

For the Tzatziki Sauce:
• 1 cup plain Greek yogurt
• 1/2 cucumber, peeled, seeded, and grated
• 1 tbsp lemon juice
• 1 clove garlic, minced
• 1 tbsp chopped fresh dill
• Salt and pepper to taste

Instructions:

1. Preheat your oven to 375°F. Line a baking sheet with parchment paper.

2. In a food processor, combine the chickpeas, cauliflower rice (or brown rice), parsley, lemon juice, cumin, garlic powder, cayenne (if using), salt, and pepper. Pulse until the mixture is well combined but still has some texture.

3. Scoop the falafel mixture by the tablespoonful and shape into small patties, about 1•inch thick. Place the falafel patties on the prepared baking sheet.

4. Bake the falafel for 15•20 minutes, flipping halfway, until golden brown and crispy.

5. While the falafel is baking, make the tzatziki sauce. In a small bowl, mix together the Greek yogurt, grated cucumber, lemon juice, garlic, dill, salt, and pepper.

6. Serve the baked falafel warm, with the tzatziki sauce on the side.

70. Grilled lamb kebabs with vegetables

Ingredient:

- 1 lb lean lamb, cut into 1•inch cubes
- 1 red bell pepper, cut into 1•inch pieces
- 1 zucchini, cut into 1•inch pieces
- 1 red onion, cut into 1•inch pieces
- 2 tbsp olive oil
- 1 tsp dried oregano
- 1 tsp garlic powder
- Salt and pepper to taste
- Lemon wedges for serving (optional)

Instructions:

1. Preheat your grill or grill pan to medium•high heat.

2. In a large bowl, combine the lamb cubes, bell pepper, zucchini, and onion. Drizzle with the olive oil and sprinkle with the oregano, garlic powder, salt, and pepper. Toss to coat the ingredients evenly.

3. Thread the lamb and vegetables onto metal or wooden skewers, alternating the ingredients.

4. Grill the kebabs for 10•12 minutes, turning occasionally, until the lamb is cooked through and the vegetables are tender. Serve the grilled lamb kebabs warm, with lemon wedges on the side if desired.

Tips:

- Use lean lamb to keep the fat and calories low.

- Cut the vegetables into similar•sized pieces to ensure even cooking.

- Stick to 2•3 kebab skewers per serving to avoid overeating.

- Pair the kebabs with a side salad or roasted cauliflower for a complete post•op friendly meal.

- If using wooden skewers, soak them in water for 30 minutes before assembling the kebabs to prevent them from burning.

71. Chicken souvlaki with tzatziki sauce

Ingredient:

• 1 lb lean ground beef or ground turkey
• 1/2 cup cooked cauliflower rice (or cooked brown rice)
• 1/2 cup finely chopped onion
• 1 egg, lightly beaten
• 2 tbsp tomato paste
• 1 tsp Worcestershire sauce
• 1 tsp dried oregano
• 1/2 tsp garlic powder
• Salt and pepper to taste

Instructions:

1. Preheat your oven to 375°F. Lightly grease a 9x5•inch loaf pan.

2. In a large bowl, combine the ground beef or turkey, cauliflower rice (or brown rice), onion, egg, tomato paste, Worcestershire sauce, oregano, garlic powder, salt, and pepper. Mix until well incorporated.

3. Transfer the meatloaf mixture to the prepared loaf pan, gently pressing it into an even layer.

4. Bake the meatloaf for 45•55 minutes, or until the internal temperature reaches 165°F.

5. Let the meatloaf rest for 5•10 minutes before slicing and serving.

Tips:

• Use lean ground beef or turkey to keep the fat and calories low.

• Opt for cauliflower rice or brown rice to provide fiber and nutrients.

• Stick to a 4•6 oz portion of the meatloaf to avoid overeating.

• Serve the meatloaf with roasted vegetables or a side salad for a complete post•op friendly meal.

• You can also make individual meatloaf portions in a muffin tin for easier portion control.

• For added moisture, you can mix in a small amount of low•fat milk or broth.

72. Beef and vegetable kabobs

Ingredient:

• 1 lb lean beef sirloin or tenderloin, cut into 1•inch cubes
• 1 red bell pepper, cut into 1•inch pieces
• 1 zucchini, cut into 1•inch pieces
• 1 red onion, cut into 1•inch pieces
• 2 tbsp olive oil
• 1 tsp dried oregano
• 1 tsp garlic powder
• Salt and pepper to taste
• Lemon wedges for serving (optional)

Instructions:

1. Preheat your grill or grill pan to medium•high heat.

2. In a large bowl, combine the beef cubes, bell pepper, zucchini, and onion. Drizzle with the olive oil and sprinkle with the oregano, garlic powder, salt, and pepper. Toss to coat the ingredients evenly.

3. Thread the beef and vegetables onto metal or wooden skewers, alternating the ingredients.

4. Grill the kabobs for 10•12 minutes, turning occasionally, until the beef is cooked through and the vegetables are tender.

5. Serve the grilled beef and vegetable kabobs warm, with lemon wedges on the side if desired.

Tips:

• Use lean beef sirloin or tenderloin to keep the fat and calories low.
• Cut the vegetables into similar•sized pieces to ensure even cooking.
• Stick to 2•3 kabob skewers per serving to avoid overeating.
• Pair the kabobs with a side salad or roasted cauliflower for a complete post•op friendly meal.
• If using wooden skewers, soak them in water for 30 minutes before assembling the kabobs to prevent them from burning.

73. Meatloaf made with lean ground beef or turkey

Ingredient:

- 1 lb lean ground beef or ground turkey
- 1/2 cup cooked cauliflower rice (or cooked brown rice)
- 1/2 cup finely chopped onion
- 1 egg, lightly beaten
- 2 tbsp tomato paste
- 1 tsp Worcestershire sauce
- 1 tsp dried oregano
- 1/2 tsp garlic powder
- Salt and pepper to taste

Instructions:

1. Preheat your oven to 375°F. Lightly grease a 9x5•inch loaf pan.

2. In a large bowl, combine the ground beef or turkey, cauliflower rice (or brown rice), onion, egg, tomato paste, Worcestershire sauce, oregano, garlic powder, salt, and pepper. Mix until well incorporated.

3. Transfer the meatloaf mixture to the prepared loaf pan, gently pressing it into an even layer.

4. Bake the meatloaf for 45•55 minutes, or until the internal temperature reaches 165°F.

5. Let the meatloaf rest for 5•10 minutes before slicing and serving.

Tips:

- Use lean ground beef or turkey to keep the fat and calories low.

- Opt for cauliflower rice or brown rice to provide fiber and nutrients.

- Stick to a 4•6 oz portion of the meatloaf to avoid overeating.

- Serve the meatloaf with roasted vegetables or a side salad for a complete post•op friendly meal.

- You can also make individual meatloaf portions in a muffin tin for easier portion control.

- For added moisture, you can mix in a small amount of low•fat milk or broth.

74. Shepherd's pie with lean ground beef or turkey

Ingredient:

For the Filling:
• 1 lb lean ground beef or ground turkey
• 1 onion, diced
• 2 carrots, peeled and diced
• 2 celery stalks, diced
• 2 cloves garlic, minced
• 1 tbsp tomato paste
• 1 tsp Worcestershire sauce
• 1 tsp dried thyme
• 1 cup low•sodium beef or chicken broth
• Salt and pepper to taste

For the Topping:
• 1 lb cauliflower, cut into florets (or 2 cups cooked mashed potatoes)
• 2 tbsp low•fat milk or unsweetened almond milk
• 2 tbsp grated Parmesan cheese
• Salt and pepper to taste

Instructions:
1. Preheat your oven to 375°F. Grease a 9x13•inch baking dish.

2. In a large skillet over medium•high heat, cook the ground beef or turkey, breaking it up as it cooks, until browned, about 5•7 minutes. Drain any excess fat.

3. Add the onion, carrots, celery, and garlic to the skillet. Cook for 5•7 minutes, until the vegetables are softened.

4. Stir in the tomato paste, Worcestershire sauce, thyme, and broth. Simmer for 10•15 minutes, until the sauce has thickened. Season with salt and pepper to taste.

5. In a food processor or blender, puree the cauliflower florets (or mash the potatoes) with the milk and Parmesan cheese. Season with salt and pepper.

6. Spread the beef or turkey mixture in the prepared baking dish. Top with the cauliflower (or potato) topping, spreading it evenly.

7. Bake for 25•30 minutes, until the topping is lightly browned and the filling is bubbling. Let the shepherd's pie cool for 5•10 minutes before serving.

75. Spaghetti with meat sauce (using lean ground beef or turkey)

Ingredient:

- 8 oz cooked spaghetti squash or zucchini noodles
- 1 lb lean ground beef or ground turkey
- 1 onion, diced
- 2 cloves garlic, minced
- 1 (28 oz) can crushed tomatoes
- 2 tbsp tomato paste
- 1 tsp dried oregano
- 1 tsp dried basil
- Salt and pepper to taste
- 2 tbsp grated Parmesan cheese (optional)

Instructions:

1. In a large skillet over medium•high heat, cook the ground beef or turkey, breaking it up as it cooks, until browned, about 5•7 minutes. Drain any excess fat.

2. Add the diced onion and minced garlic to the skillet. Cook for 3•5 minutes, until the onion is translucent.

3. Stir in the crushed tomatoes, tomato paste, oregano, and basil. Season with salt and pepper to taste.

4. Reduce the heat to low and let the sauce simmer for 15•20 minutes, stirring occasionally, to allow the flavors to meld.

5. While the sauce is simmering, prepare the spaghetti squash or zucchini noodles according to package instructions.

6. Serve the meat sauce over the cooked spaghetti squash or zucchini noodles. Top with a sprinkle of grated Parmesan cheese, if desired.

Tips:
- Use lean ground beef or turkey to keep the fat and calories low.
- Opt for spaghetti squash or zucchini noodles to reduce the carb content.
- Stick to a 1•cup portion of the spaghetti and meat sauce to avoid overeating.
- Pair the dish with a side salad or roasted vegetables for a complete post•op friendly meal.
- You can also make the meat sauce in advance and freeze it for easy reheating on busy days.

76. Lasagna with cottage cheese and lean ground beef or turkey

Ingredient:

- 1 lb lean ground beef or ground turkey
- 1 onion, diced
- 2 cloves garlic, minced
- 1 (24 oz) jar low•sugar marinara sauce
- 1 (15 oz) container low•fat cottage cheese
- 1 egg
- 1/4 cup grated Parmesan cheese
- 2 cups shredded low•fat mozzarella cheese
- 8 no•boil lasagna noodles

Instructions:

1. Preheat your oven to 375°F. Grease a 9x13•inch baking dish.

2. In a large skillet over medium•high heat, cook the ground beef or turkey, breaking it up as it cooks, until browned, about 5•7 minutes. Drain any excess fat.

3. Add the onion and garlic to the skillet and cook for 3•5 minutes, until the onion is translucent.

4. Stir in the marinara sauce and simmer for 5•10 minutes.

5. In a medium bowl, mix together the cottage cheese, egg, and Parmesan cheese.

6. Spread 1 cup of the meat sauce in the bottom of the prepared baking dish. Arrange 4 lasagna noodles over the sauce. Spread half of the cottage cheese mixture over the noodles, then top with 1 cup of the meat sauce and 1/2 cup of the mozzarella cheese.

7. Repeat the layers of noodles, cottage cheese, meat sauce, and mozzarella cheese.

8. Cover the dish with foil and bake for 30 minutes. Remove the foil and bake for an additional 15•20 minutes, until the cheese is melted and bubbly.

9. Let the lasagna cool for 10•15 minutes before serving.

77. Stuffed shells with ricotta and spinach

Ingredient:

- 12 jumbo pasta shells
- 1 cup part•skim ricotta cheese
- 1 cup chopped fresh spinach
- 1/4 cup grated Parmesan cheese
- 1 egg, lightly beaten
- 1 tsp dried oregano
- 1/2 tsp garlic powder
- Salt and pepper to taste
- 1 cup marinara sauce
- 1/2 cup shredded low•fat mozzarella cheese

Instructions:

1. Preheat your oven to 375°F. Grease a 9x13•inch baking dish.

2. Cook the pasta shells according to package instructions until al dente. Drain and set aside.

3. In a medium bowl, mix together the ricotta cheese, spinach, Parmesan cheese, egg, oregano, garlic powder, salt, and pepper.

4. Stuff each cooked pasta shell with a heaping tablespoon of the ricotta•spinach mixture.

5. Spread 1/2 cup of the marinara sauce in the bottom of the prepared baking dish. Arrange the stuffed shells in a single layer on top of the sauce.

6. Pour the remaining 1/2 cup of marinara sauce over the stuffed shells, then sprinkle the shredded mozzarella cheese on top.

7. Bake the stuffed shells for 20•25 minutes, until the cheese is melted and bubbly. Let the stuffed shells cool for 5•10 minutes before serving.

Tips:
- Use part•skim ricotta cheese to keep the fat and calories lower.
- Opt for fresh spinach over frozen to avoid excess moisture.
- Stick to 2•3 stuffed shells per serving to avoid overeating.
- Pair the stuffed shells with a side salad or roasted vegetables for a complete post•op friendly meal.
- You can also make the stuffed shells in advance and freeze them for easy reheating on busy days.

78. Baked ziti with lean ground beef or turkey

Ingredient:

- 8 oz zucchini noodles or shirataki noodles
- 1 lb lean ground beef or ground turkey
- 1 onion, diced
- 2 cloves garlic, minced
- 1 (24 oz) jar low·sugar marinara sauce
- 1 cup low·fat ricotta cheese
- 1/4 cup grated Parmesan cheese
- 1 egg, lightly beaten
- 1 tsp dried oregano
- 1/2 tsp dried basil
- Salt and pepper to taste
- 1 cup shredded low·fat mozzarella cheese

Instructions:

1. Preheat your oven to 375°F. Grease a 9x13·inch baking dish.

2. Prepare the zucchini noodles or shirataki noodles according to package instructions. Drain and set aside.

3. In a large skillet over medium·high heat, cook the ground beef or turkey, breaking it up as it cooks, until browned, about 5·7 minutes. Drain any excess fat.

4. Add the diced onion and minced garlic to the skillet. Cook for 3·5 minutes, until the onion is translucent.

5. Stir in the marinara sauce and simmer for 5·10 minutes.

6. In a medium bowl, mix together the ricotta cheese, Parmesan cheese, egg, oregano, basil, salt, and pepper.

7. Spread 1/2 cup of the meat sauce in the bottom of the prepared baking dish. Layer half of the zucchini or shirataki noodles over the sauce, then top with half of the ricotta cheese mixture and half of the remaining meat sauce.

8. Repeat the layers of noodles, ricotta cheese, and meat sauce. Top the casserole with the shredded mozzarella cheese. Bake the baked ziti for 25·30 minutes, until the cheese is melted and bubbly. Let the baked ziti cool for 10·15 minutes before serving.

79. Chicken parmesan with low•fat cheese

Ingredient:

• 4 boneless, skinless chicken breasts, pounded thin
• 1/2 cup whole wheat panko breadcrumbs
• 1/4 cup grated Parmesan cheese
• 1 tsp dried oregano
• 1/2 tsp garlic powder
• Salt and pepper to taste
• 1 egg, beaten
• 1 cup marinara sauce
• 1 cup shredded low•fat mozzarella cheese

Instructions:

1. Preheat your oven to 400°F. Lightly grease a baking sheet or oven•safe dish.

2. In a shallow bowl, mix together the panko breadcrumbs, Parmesan cheese, oregano, garlic powder, salt, and pepper.

3. Dip the chicken breasts into the beaten egg, then coat them in the breadcrumb mixture, pressing gently to adhere.

4. Arrange the breaded chicken breasts in a single layer on the prepared baking sheet or dish.

5. Bake the chicken for 15•20 minutes, or until it's cooked through and the breading is golden brown.

6. Remove the chicken from the oven and top each piece with 1/4 cup of the marinara sauce and 1/4 cup of the shredded mozzarella cheese.

7. Return the chicken to the oven and bake for an additional 5•10 minutes, until the cheese is melted and bubbly.

8. Let the chicken parmesan cool for 5 minutes before serving.

80. Eggplant parmesan

Ingredient:

• 1 medium eggplant, sliced into 1/4·inch thick rounds
• 1 egg, beaten
• 1/2 cup grated Parmesan cheese
• 1/2 cup panko breadcrumbs
• 1 tsp dried oregano
• 1/2 tsp garlic powder
• Salt and pepper to taste
• 1 cup marinara sauce
• 1 cup shredded low·fat mozzarella cheese

Instructions:

1. Preheat your oven to 375°F. Lightly grease a baking sheet.

2. In a shallow bowl, beat the egg. In another shallow bowl, mix together the Parmesan cheese, panko breadcrumbs, oregano, garlic powder, salt, and pepper.

3. Dip the eggplant slices into the beaten egg, then coat them in the Parmesan·breadcrumb mixture, pressing gently to adhere.

4. Arrange the breaded eggplant slices in a single layer on the prepared baking sheet.

5. Bake the eggplant for 15·20 minutes, flipping halfway, until golden brown and crispy.

6. Spread 1/2 cup of the marinara sauce in the bottom of a baking dish. Arrange the baked eggplant slices in a single layer over the sauce.

7. Top the eggplant with the remaining 1/2 cup of marinara sauce and the shredded mozzarella cheese.

8. Bake the eggplant parmesan for an additional 15·20 minutes, until the cheese is melted and bubbly. Let the eggplant parmesan cool for 5·10 minutes before serving.

Tips:
• Use panko breadcrumbs instead of regular breadcrumbs for a lighter, crispier coating.
• Stick to a 1·2 slice portion of the eggplant parmesan to avoid overeating.
• Pair the eggplant parmesan with a side salad or roasted vegetables for a complete post·op friendly meal.

81. Ratatouille (vegetable stew)

Ingredient:

- 1 medium eggplant, diced
- 1 zucchini, diced
- 1 yellow squash, diced
- 1 red bell pepper, diced
- 1 onion, diced
- 3 cloves garlic, minced
- 2 tbsp olive oil
- 1 (14 oz) can diced tomatoes
- 2 tbsp tomato paste
- 1 tsp dried thyme
- 1 tsp dried oregano
- Salt and pepper to taste
- 2 tbsp chopped fresh basil (optional)

Instructions:

1. In a large skillet or Dutch oven, heat the olive oil over medium heat.

2. Add the diced eggplant, zucchini, yellow squash, bell pepper, onion, and garlic. Sauté for 8•10 minutes, stirring occasionally, until the vegetables are starting to soften.

3. Stir in the diced tomatoes, tomato paste, thyme, and oregano. Season with salt and pepper to taste.

4. Reduce the heat to low, cover the pot, and simmer for 20•25 minutes, stirring occasionally, until the vegetables are very tender.

5. Remove the lid and continue simmering for 5•10 minutes to allow the flavors to meld and the sauce to thicken slightly.

6. Stir in the chopped fresh basil, if using. Serve the ratatouille warm, either on its own or over a bed of cauliflower rice or zucchini noodles.

Tips:
- Use a variety of colorful vegetables to maximize the nutrient content.
- Opt for fresh, in•season produce for the best flavor.
- Stick to a 1•cup portion of the ratatouille to avoid overeating.
- Pair the ratatouille with a protein•rich side, such as grilled chicken or shrimp, for a complete post•op friendly meal.
- This dish can be made in advance and reheated, making it a great option for meal prep.

82. Frittata with vegetables and low•fat cheese

Ingredient:

- 6 eggs
- 1/4 cup low•fat milk
- 1/4 tsp salt
- 1/4 tsp black pepper
- 1 cup chopped vegetables (such as spinach, bell peppers, onions, mushrooms)
- 1/2 cup shredded low•fat cheddar or mozzarella cheese

Instructions:

1. Preheat your oven to 375°F (190°C).

2. In a medium bowl, whisk together the eggs, milk, salt, and black pepper until well combined.

3. Spray a 9•inch oven•safe non•stick skillet with cooking spray and place it over medium heat.

4. Add the chopped vegetables to the skillet and sauté for 2•3 minutes, until they start to soften.

5. Pour the egg mixture over the vegetables and let it cook for 2•3 minutes, until the edges start to set.

6. Sprinkle the shredded low•fat cheese over the top of the frittata.

7. Transfer the skillet to the preheated oven and bake for 12•15 minutes, or until the frittata is set and the cheese is melted and bubbly.

8. Remove the frittata from the oven and let it cool for a few minutes before slicing and serving.

This frittata is a great source of protein, fiber, and nutrients, and the low•fat cheese helps keep the fat content in check, making it a suitable option for those following a post•gastric bypass diet. Enjoy!

83. Quiche with spinach and low•fat cheese

Ingredient:

• 1 pre•baked 9•inch pie crust (use a low•carb or gluten•free crust if desired)
• 1 tbsp olive oil
• 1 onion, diced
• 3 cups fresh spinach, chopped
• 6 eggs
• 1 cup low•fat milk
• 1/2 cup shredded low•fat cheddar or Swiss cheese
• 2 tbsp grated Parmesan cheese
• 1/2 tsp dried thyme
• Salt and pepper to taste

Instructions:

1. Preheat your oven to 375°F.

2. In a skillet over medium heat, heat the olive oil. Add the diced onion and sauté for 3•5 minutes until translucent.

3. Add the chopped spinach to the skillet and cook for 2•3 minutes until wilted. Remove from heat and let cool slightly.

4. In a large bowl, whisk together the eggs and milk. Stir in the sautéed spinach and onion mixture, the shredded low•fat cheese, Parmesan cheese, thyme, salt, and pepper.

5. Pour the egg mixture into the pre•baked pie crust.

6. Bake the quiche for 35•40 minutes, or until the center is set and the top is lightly golden.

7. Allow the quiche to cool for 10•15 minutes before slicing and serving.

Tips:

• Use a pre•baked low•carb or gluten•free pie crust to keep the carbs low.
• Opt for low•fat cheese to reduce the overall fat and calorie content.
• Stick to a 1•2 slice portion of the quiche to avoid overeating.
• Pair the quiche with a side salad or roasted vegetables for a complete post•op friendly meal.
• You can also make individual quiche cups in a muffin tin for easier portion control.

84. Eggs Benedict with Canadian bacon and light hollandaise sauce

Ingredient:

• 4 eggs
• 4 slices of Canadian bacon
• 2 English muffins, split in half
• For the Hollandaise Sauce:
• 2 egg yolks
• 2 tbsp lemon juice
• 1/4 cup low•fat milk
• 1 tbsp unsalted butter, melted
• 1/4 tsp salt
• 1/8 tsp white pepper

Instructions:

1. Prepare the hollandaise sauce:
   • In a small saucepan, whisk together the egg yolks and lemon juice until well combined.
   • Place the saucepan over low heat and slowly whisk in the milk. Cook, whisking constantly, until the mixture thickens slightly, about 2•3 minutes.
   • Remove the saucepan from the heat and whisk in the melted butter. Season with salt and white pepper.
   • Keep the hollandaise sauce warm while you prepare the rest of the dish.

2. Poach the eggs:
   • Bring a large pot of water to a gentle simmer. Crack each egg individually into a small bowl or cup, then gently slide the eggs into the simmering water.
   • Poach the eggs for 3•4 minutes, or until the whites are set and the yolks are still runny.
   • Remove the poached eggs from the water using a slotted spoon and set aside.

3. Cook the Canadian bacon:
   • In a skillet over medium heat, cook the Canadian bacon slices for 2•3 minutes per side, or until heated through and slightly crispy.

4. Assemble the Eggs Benedict:
   • Place the English muffin halves on plates and top each half with a slice of Canadian bacon.
   • Carefully place a poached egg on top of the Canadian bacon.
   • Drizzle the warm hollandaise sauce over the top of the eggs.

85. Huevos rancheros with black beans and salsa

Ingredient:

• 4 eggs
• 1 (15 oz) can black beans, rinsed and drained
• 1/2 cup low•fat or non•fat plain Greek yogurt
• 1/2 cup salsa (look for a low•sugar variety)
• 2 tbsp chopped fresh cilantro
• 1/4 tsp ground cumin
• Salt and pepper to taste
• Cooking spray

Instructions:

1. In a small saucepan, heat the black beans over medium heat, stirring occasionally, until heated through, about 5 minutes. Remove from heat and keep warm.

2. In a non•stick skillet coated with cooking spray, cook the eggs over medium heat until the whites are set and the yolks are still runny, about 2•3 minutes.

3. To serve, place the warm black beans on a plate. Top with the cooked eggs.

4. In a small bowl, mix together the Greek yogurt, salsa, cilantro, and cumin. Season with salt and pepper to taste.

5. Spoon the yogurt•salsa mixture over the eggs and black beans.

Serve immediately and enjoy your post•gastric bypass friendly Huevos Rancheros!

This dish is a great source of protein, fiber, and healthy fats, and the Greek yogurt and salsa provide a flavorful and low•calorie topping. The black beans are a good source of fiber and nutrients, making this a well•balanced meal for those following a post•gastric bypass diet.

86. Breakfast burrito with scrambled eggs, black beans, and salsa

Ingredient:

• 4 eggs, beaten
• 1/4 cup low•fat milk
• 1/4 tsp salt
• 1/4 tsp black pepper
• 1 (15 oz) can black beans, rinsed and drained
• 1/2 cup salsa (look for a low•sugar variety)
• 2 small whole wheat tortillas or low•carb wraps

Instructions:

1. In a non•stick skillet coated with cooking spray, scramble the eggs with the milk, salt, and black pepper over medium heat, stirring frequently, until the eggs are cooked through, about 3•4 minutes. Remove from heat and set aside.

2. In a small saucepan, heat the black beans over medium heat, stirring occasionally, until heated through, about 5 minutes. Remove from heat and keep warm.

3. To assemble the burritos:

  • Lay the tortillas or wraps on a flat surface.

  • Divide the scrambled eggs evenly between the two tortillas, placing them in the center.

  • Top the eggs with the warm black beans, followed by the salsa.

  • Fold the bottom of the tortilla up over the filling, then fold in the sides and continue rolling up tightly to create a burrito.

Serve the breakfast burritos immediately and enjoy!

This breakfast burrito is a great option for those following a post•gastric bypass diet. The scrambled eggs provide protein, the black beans offer fiber and nutrients, and the salsa adds flavor without too many additional calories or carbs. The whole wheat tortilla or low•carb wrap helps keep the carbohydrate content in check.

87. Oatmeal with cinnamon and sliced almonds

Ingredient:

- 1/2 cup old•fashioned oats
- 1 cup unsweetened almond milk (or low•fat milk)
- 1/4 tsp ground cinnamon
- 1 tbsp sliced almonds
- 1 tsp honey (optional)

Instructions:

1. In a small saucepan, combine the oats and almond milk (or low•fat milk).

2. Bring the mixture to a simmer over medium heat, stirring occasionally, until the oats are tender and the liquid is absorbed, about 5•7 minutes.

3. Remove the oatmeal from the heat and stir in the ground cinnamon.

4. Transfer the oatmeal to a bowl and top with the sliced almonds.

5. If desired, drizzle the oatmeal with a small amount of honey for a touch of sweetness.

Serve the oatmeal warm and enjoy!

This oatmeal dish is a great option for those following a post•gastric bypass diet. Oats are a good source of fiber, which can help promote feelings of fullness and support healthy digestion. The cinnamon adds flavor without any additional calories or carbs, and the sliced almonds provide a satisfying crunch while also contributing healthy fats and protein.

Remember to adjust the portion size as needed to fit your individual dietary needs and preferences. Enjoy this nutritious and delicious breakfast!

88. Chia seed pudding with almond milk and berries

Ingredient:

- 1/4 cup chia seeds
- 1 cup unsweetened almond milk
- 1 tsp vanilla extract
- 1/4 tsp ground cinnamon
- 1 cup mixed berries (such as raspberries, blueberries, and/or strawberries)

Instructions:

1. In a medium·sized bowl, whisk together the chia seeds, almond milk, vanilla extract, and cinnamon until well combined.

2. Cover the bowl and refrigerate the chia seed mixture for at least 2 hours, or up to overnight, stirring occasionally, until it has thickened to a pudding·like consistency.

3. When ready to serve, divide the chia seed pudding evenly between two bowls or jars.

4. Top each serving with 1/2 cup of the mixed berries.

5. Serve chilled and enjoy!

This chia seed pudding is a great option for a post·gastric bypass breakfast or snack. Chia seeds are high in fiber, protein, and healthy omega·3 fatty acids, which can help support overall health and digestion. The almond milk provides a creamy texture without too many additional calories or carbs, and the berries add natural sweetness and antioxidants.

Feel free to adjust the amount of chia seeds or almond milk to achieve your desired consistency. You can also experiment with different types of berries or other toppings, such as sliced almonds or a drizzle of honey, to customize the recipe to your taste.

89. Protein pancakes with sugar•free syrup

Ingredient:

- 1/2 cup rolled oats
- 2 scoops (about 1/4 cup) unflavored or vanilla protein powder
- 1/4 cup egg whites (or 2 large eggs)
- 1/4 cup unsweetened almond milk
- 1 tsp baking powder
- 1/4 tsp ground cinnamon
- 1/4 cup sugar•free maple syrup

Instructions:

1. In a blender or food processor, blend the rolled oats until they reach a flour•like consistency.

2. Add the protein powder, egg whites (or eggs), almond milk, baking powder, and cinnamon to the blender. Blend until the batter is smooth and well combined.

3. Heat a non•stick skillet or griddle over medium heat and lightly coat with cooking spray.

4. Scoop the batter onto the hot surface, using approximately 1/4 cup of batter per pancake.

5. Cook the pancakes for 2•3 minutes per side, or until they are golden brown and cooked through.

6. Serve the protein pancakes warm, drizzled with the sugar•free maple syrup.

These protein•packed pancakes are a great option for a post•gastric bypass breakfast. The oats and protein powder provide a good source of protein and fiber, while the sugar•free syrup adds sweetness without the extra calories and carbs. Feel free to top the pancakes with fresh berries or a dollop of plain Greek yogurt for added nutrition and flavor.

Remember to adjust the portion sizes as needed to fit your individual dietary needs and preferences. Enjoy this delicious and nutritious breakfast!

90. Protein waffles with sugar•free syrup

Ingredient:

• 1 cup rolled oats
• 2 scoops (about 1/4 cup) unflavored or vanilla protein powder
• 1 cup unsweetened almond milk
• 2 large eggs
• 1 tsp baking powder
• 1/4 tsp ground cinnamon
• 1/4 cup sugar•free maple syrup

Instructions:

1. Preheat your waffle iron according to the manufacturer's instructions.

2. In a blender or food processor, blend the rolled oats until they reach a flour•like consistency.

3. Add the protein powder, almond milk, eggs, baking powder, and cinnamon to the blender. Blend until the batter is smooth and well combined.

4. Lightly coat the preheated waffle iron with cooking spray.

5. Pour the batter onto the waffle iron, using about 1/2 cup of batter per waffle. Cook the waffles for 3•5 minutes, or until they are golden brown and cooked through.

6. Carefully remove the waffles from the iron and place them on a plate.

7. Serve the protein waffles warm, drizzled with the sugar•free maple syrup.

These protein•packed waffles are a great option for a post•gastric bypass breakfast. The oats and protein powder provide a good source of protein and fiber, while the sugar•free syrup adds sweetness without the extra calories and carbs. Feel free to top the waffles with fresh berries or a dollop of plain Greek yogurt for added nutrition and flavor.

Remember to adjust the portion sizes as needed to fit your individual dietary needs and preferences. Enjoy this delicious and nutritious breakfast!

91. French toast made with whole•grain bread and egg whites

Ingredient:

- 4 slices of whole•grain or whole•wheat bread
- 4 large egg whites
- 1/4 cup unsweetened almond milk
- 1 tsp vanilla extract
- 1/2 tsp ground cinnamon
- Cooking spray

Instructions:

1. In a shallow bowl, whisk together the egg whites, almond milk, vanilla extract, and cinnamon until well combined.

2. Dip each slice of bread into the egg white mixture, coating both sides evenly.

3. Heat a non•stick skillet or griddle over medium heat and lightly coat with cooking spray.

4. Cook the French toast slices for 2•3 minutes per side, or until golden brown and cooked through.

5. Serve the French toast warm, with your choice of toppings such as:
   - Fresh berries
   - A drizzle of sugar•free maple syrup
   - A sprinkle of cinnamon

This French toast recipe is a great option for a post•gastric bypass breakfast. The whole•grain bread provides fiber, while the egg whites are a lean source of protein. The almond milk and cinnamon add flavor without too many additional calories or carbs.

Remember to adjust the portion sizes as needed to fit your individual dietary needs and preferences. Enjoy this delicious and nutritious French toast!

92. Tofu scramble with vegetables

Ingredient:

- 1 block (14 oz) firm or extra•firm tofu, drained and crumbled
- 1 tbsp olive oil
- 1/2 cup diced onion
- 1/2 cup diced bell pepper
- 1 cup chopped spinach or kale
- 2 tbsp nutritional yeast
- 1 tsp ground cumin
- 1/2 tsp garlic powder
- 1/4 tsp turmeric
- Salt and black pepper to taste

Instructions:

1. Heat the olive oil in a large non•stick skillet over medium heat.

2. Add the diced onion and bell pepper to the skillet. Sauté for 3•4 minutes, or until the vegetables are softened.

3. Add the crumbled tofu to the skillet and use a spatula to break it up into smaller pieces, mimicking the texture of scrambled eggs.

4. Stir in the nutritional yeast, cumin, garlic powder, and turmeric. Cook for 2•3 minutes, stirring frequently, to allow the flavors to blend.

5. Add the chopped spinach or kale to the skillet and continue cooking for another 1•2 minutes, or until the greens are wilted.

6. Season the tofu scramble with salt and black pepper to taste.

7. Serve the tofu scramble warm, either on its own or with a side of roasted vegetables or a small portion of whole•grain toast.

This tofu scramble is a great source of plant•based protein, fiber, and essential nutrients. The vegetables add color, texture, and additional vitamins and minerals. It's a delicious and satisfying option for a post•gastric bypass breakfast or brunch.

Remember to adjust the portion sizes as needed to fit your individual dietary needs and preferences. Enjoy this nutritious and flavorful tofu scramble!

93. Egg white and vegetable frittata

Ingredient:

• 8 egg whites
• 1/2 cup diced bell pepper
• 1/2 cup diced onion
• 1/2 cup diced mushrooms
• 1/4 cup shredded low•fat cheese (such as cheddar or mozzarella)
• 2 tbsp milk or unsweetened almond milk
• Salt and pepper to taste

Instructions:

1. Preheat oven to 375°F.

2. In a medium bowl, whisk together the egg whites, milk, salt, and pepper.

3. Spray a 9•inch oven•safe skillet or pie dish with non•stick cooking spray.

4. Add the diced vegetables to the skillet and sauté over medium heat for 3•5 minutes until softened.

5. Pour the egg white mixture over the vegetables and sprinkle the shredded cheese on top.

6. Bake for 20•25 minutes, or until the frittata is set and the cheese is melted.

7. Allow to cool for 5 minutes before slicing and serving.

This frittata is high in protein from the egg whites, low in fat, and contains a variety of nutrient•dense vegetables. It can be a great option for those following a post•gastric bypass diet, as it is easy to digest and provides a balance of protein, vegetables, and a small amount of dairy. Adjust portion sizes as needed to meet your individual dietary needs.

94. Chicken and vegetable soup

Ingredient:

- 4 cups low•sodium chicken broth
- 1 lb boneless, skinless chicken breasts, diced
- 1 cup diced carrots
- 1 cup diced celery
- 1 cup diced onion
- 1 cup diced zucchini
- 1 cup diced mushrooms
- 2 cloves garlic, minced
- 1 tsp dried thyme
- 1 tsp dried parsley
- Salt and pepper to taste

Instructions:

1. In a large pot, bring the chicken broth to a boil over medium•high heat.

2. Add the diced chicken, carrots, celery, onion, zucchini, mushrooms, and garlic. Reduce heat to medium•low and simmer for 15•20 minutes, or until the vegetables are tender and the chicken is cooked through.

3. Stir in the dried thyme and parsley. Season with salt and pepper to taste.

4. Serve hot.

This soup is a great option for those following a post•gastric bypass diet as it is low in calories, high in protein from the chicken, and packed with a variety of nutrient•dense vegetables. The broth•based soup is also easy to digest and can help to keep you hydrated. Adjust portion sizes as needed to meet your individual dietary needs.

95. Beef and barley soup

Ingredient:

- 1 lb lean beef stew meat, cut into 1·inch cubes
- 1 tbsp olive oil
- 1 onion, diced
- 3 carrots, peeled and diced
- 3 celery stalks, diced
- 4 cups low·sodium beef broth
- 1 cup pearl barley
- 2 bay leaves
- 1 tsp dried thyme
- Salt and pepper to taste

Instructions:

1. In a large pot or Dutch oven, heat the olive oil over medium·high heat. Add the beef cubes and brown on all sides, about 5 minutes total. Remove the beef from the pot and set aside.

2. Add the onion, carrots, and celery to the pot and sauté for 5·7 minutes, until the vegetables are softened.

3. Add the beef broth, pearl barley, bay leaves, and thyme. Bring the mixture to a boil, then reduce the heat to low, cover, and simmer for 45·60 minutes, or until the barley is tender.

4. Add the browned beef back to the pot and season with salt and pepper to taste. Serve hot.

This beef and barley soup is a great option for those following a post·gastric bypass diet as it is high in protein from the beef, contains fiber·rich barley, and is packed with nutrient·dense vegetables. The broth·based soup is also easy to digest. Adjust portion sizes as needed to meet your individual dietary needs.

96. Split pea soup with ham

Ingredient:

- 1 lb dried split peas, rinsed
- 6 cups low•sodium chicken or vegetable broth
- 1 cup diced ham
- 1 onion, diced
- 2 carrots, peeled and diced
- 2 celery stalks, diced
- 2 cloves garlic, minced
- 1 tsp dried thyme
- Salt and pepper to taste

Instructions:

1. In a large pot, combine the rinsed split peas and broth. Bring to a boil over high heat.

2. Reduce heat to medium•low, cover, and simmer for 45•60 minutes, stirring occasionally, until the peas are very soft.

3. Add the diced ham, onion, carrots, celery, and garlic. Simmer for an additional 15•20 minutes, until the vegetables are tender.

4. Stir in the dried thyme and season with salt and pepper to taste. Serve hot.

This split pea soup is a great option for those following a post•gastric bypass diet for a few reasons:

• The split peas are a good source of protein and fiber, which can help promote feelings of fullness.

• The ham provides additional protein without a lot of fat.

• The broth•based soup is easy to digest and hydrating.

• The vegetables add important vitamins, minerals, and antioxidants.

Adjust portion sizes as needed to meet your individual dietary needs. This soup can also be pureed for a smoother texture if desired.

97. Turkey chili with beans

Ingredient:

- 1 lb ground turkey
- 1 onion, diced
- 3 cloves garlic, minced
- 2 bell peppers, diced
- 2 cans (15 oz each) low•sodium black beans, rinsed and drained
- 1 can (15 oz) low•sodium kidney beans, rinsed and drained
- 1 can (28 oz) low•sodium diced tomatoes
- 2 tbsp chili powder
- 1 tsp ground cumin
- 1 tsp dried oregano
- 1/2 tsp cayenne pepper (optional)
- Salt and pepper to taste

Instructions:

1. In a large pot or Dutch oven, cook the ground turkey over medium•high heat until browned and crumbled, about 5•7 minutes. Drain any excess fat.

2. Add the diced onion, garlic, and bell peppers to the pot. Sauté for 5•7 minutes until the vegetables are softened.

3. Stir in the black beans, kidney beans, diced tomatoes, chili powder, cumin, oregano, and cayenne (if using). Season with salt and pepper.

4. Bring the chili to a simmer, then reduce heat to low and let it cook for 20•30 minutes, stirring occasionally, until the flavors have melded.

5. Serve hot, garnished with any desired toppings like diced avocado, low•fat shredded cheese, or chopped cilantro.

This turkey chili is a great option for those following a post•gastric bypass diet for a few reasons:

- The lean ground turkey provides protein without a lot of fat.
- The beans add fiber and additional protein.
- The vegetables provide important nutrients and antioxidants.
- The chili is a hearty, filling dish that is easy to digest.

98. White chicken chili

Ingredient:

- 1 lb boneless, skinless chicken breasts, diced
- 1 onion, diced
- 3 cloves garlic, minced
- 2 cans (15 oz each) low·sodium white beans, rinsed and drained
- 1 can (4 oz) diced green chiles
- 4 cups low·sodium chicken broth
- 1 tsp ground cumin
- 1 tsp dried oregano
- 1/2 tsp ground coriander
- 1/4 tsp cayenne pepper (optional)
- Salt and pepper to taste
- Chopped cilantro for garnish (optional)

Instructions:

1. In a large pot or Dutch oven, cook the diced chicken over medium·high heat until no longer pink, about 5·7 minutes. Remove chicken from pot and set aside.

2. Add the diced onion to the pot and sauté for 3·5 minutes until translucent. Add the minced garlic and sauté for 1 minute more.

3. Stir in the white beans, diced green chiles, chicken broth, cumin, oregano, coriander, and cayenne (if using). Season with salt and pepper.

4. Bring the chili to a simmer, then reduce heat to low and let it cook for 15·20 minutes, stirring occasionally.

5. Add the cooked chicken back to the pot and simmer for 5 more minutes to allow the flavors to meld. Serve hot, garnished with chopped cilantro if desired.

This white chicken chili is a great option for those following a post·gastric bypass diet for a few reasons:

- The lean chicken provides protein without a lot of fat.
- The white beans add fiber and additional protein.
- The broth·based chili is easy to digest.
- The spices and herbs add flavor without a lot of added sugar or sodium.

99. Vegetarian chili with beans and vegetables

Ingredient:

- 2 cans (15 oz each) low•sodium black beans, rinsed and drained
- 1 can (15 oz) low•sodium kidney beans, rinsed and drained
- 1 can (28 oz) low•sodium diced tomatoes
- 1 onion, diced
- 2 bell peppers, diced
- 2 carrots, peeled and diced
- 2 celery stalks, diced
- 3 cloves garlic, minced
- 2 tbsp chili powder
- 1 tsp ground cumin
- 1 tsp dried oregano
- 1/2 tsp cayenne pepper (optional)
- Salt and pepper to taste
- Chopped cilantro for garnish (optional)

Instructions:

1. In a large pot or Dutch oven, sauté the diced onion, bell peppers, carrots, and celery over medium heat for 5•7 minutes until softened.

2. Add the minced garlic and sauté for 1 minute more.

3. Stir in the black beans, kidney beans, diced tomatoes, chili powder, cumin, oregano, and cayenne (if using). Season with salt and pepper.

4. Bring the chili to a simmer, then reduce heat to low and let it cook for 20•30 minutes, stirring occasionally, to allow the flavors to meld.

5. Serve hot, garnished with chopped cilantro if desired.

Adjust portion sizes as needed to meet your individual dietary needs. You can also use low•sodium canned beans and tomatoes to further reduce the sodium content.

100. Shrimp and vegetable gumbo

Ingredient:

• 1 lb raw shrimp, peeled and deveined
• 2 tbsp olive oil
• 1 onion, diced
• 2 celery stalks, diced
• 1 bell pepper, diced
• 3 cloves garlic, minced
• 4 cups low•sodium chicken or vegetable broth
• 1 (14.5 oz) can diced tomatoes
• 1 cup sliced okra (fresh or frozen)
• 1 tsp smoked paprika
• 1 tsp dried thyme
• 1/2 tsp cayenne pepper (optional)
• Salt and pepper to taste
• Chopped parsley for garnish (optional)

Instructions:

1. In a large pot or Dutch oven, heat the olive oil over medium•high heat. Add the diced onion, celery, and bell pepper. Sauté for 5•7 minutes until the vegetables are softened.

2. Add the minced garlic and sauté for 1 minute more.

3. Pour in the chicken or vegetable broth and diced tomatoes. Stir in the sliced okra, smoked paprika, thyme, and cayenne (if using). Season with salt and pepper.

4. Bring the gumbo to a simmer, then reduce heat to medium•low and let it cook for 15•20 minutes, stirring occasionally.

5. Add the raw shrimp to the pot and cook for 5•7 minutes more, until the shrimp are opaque and cooked through.. Serve hot, garnished with chopped parsley if desired.

This shrimp and vegetable gumbo is a great option for those following a post•gastric bypass diet for a few reasons:

• The shrimp provides lean protein.
• The vegetables add important nutrients and fiber.
• The broth•based dish is easy to digest.
• The spices and herbs add flavor without a lot of added sugar or sodium.

101. Jambalaya with chicken and turkey sausage

Ingredient:

• 1 lb boneless, skinless chicken breasts, diced
• 1 lb turkey sausage, sliced into rounds
• 1 onion, diced
• 1 bell pepper, diced
• 2 celery stalks, diced
• 3 garlic cloves, minced
• 1 (14.5 oz) can diced tomatoes
• 1 cup low•sodium chicken broth
• 1 cup uncooked brown rice
• 1 tsp smoked paprika
• 1 tsp dried thyme
• 1/2 tsp cayenne pepper (optional)
• Salt and pepper to taste

Instructions:

1. In a large pot or Dutch oven, cook the chicken and turkey sausage over medium•high heat until browned, about 5•7 minutes. Remove from pot and set aside.

2. Add the onion, bell pepper, celery, and garlic to the pot. Sauté for 5•7 minutes until vegetables are softened.

3. Stir in the diced tomatoes, chicken broth, brown rice, smoked paprika, thyme, and cayenne (if using). Season with salt and pepper.

4. Bring the mixture to a boil, then reduce heat to low, cover, and simmer for 25•30 minutes, until the rice is tender.

5. Add the cooked chicken and sausage back to the pot and stir to combine. Serve hot.

This jambalaya is a great option for those following a post•gastric bypass diet for a few reasons:

• The lean chicken and turkey sausage provide protein without a lot of fat.
• The brown rice is a whole grain that provides fiber.
• The vegetables add important nutrients and antioxidants.
• The broth•based dish is easy to digest.

102. Stuffed acorn squash with quinoa and vegetables

Ingredient:

• 2 small acorn squash, halved and seeds removed
• 1 cup cooked quinoa
• 1 lb ground turkey or lean ground beef
• 1 onion, diced
• 2 cloves garlic, minced
• 1 cup diced bell pepper
• 1 cup diced zucchini
• 1 tsp dried thyme
• 1 tsp dried oregano
• Salt and pepper to taste
• 1/4 cup shredded low•fat mozzarella cheese (optional)

Instructions:

1. Preheat oven to 400°F. Place the acorn squash halves cut•side down on a baking sheet. Bake for 30•40 minutes, until tender when pierced with a fork.

2. While the squash is baking, in a large skillet, cook the ground turkey or beef over medium•high heat until browned and crumbled, about 5•7 minutes. Drain any excess fat.

3. Add the diced onion, garlic, bell pepper, and zucchini to the skillet. Sauté for 5•7 minutes until the vegetables are softened.

4. Stir in the cooked quinoa, dried thyme, and dried oregano. Season with salt and pepper.

5. Once the squash is tender, carefully scoop out the flesh, leaving about 1/2 inch of the squash intact to create a "boat". Mash the squash flesh and stir it into the quinoa and vegetable mixture.

6. Spoon the quinoa and vegetable stuffing back into the squash boats. If using, sprinkle the shredded mozzarella cheese over the top.

7. Return the stuffed squash halves to the oven and bake for an additional 10•15 minutes, until the cheese is melted. Serve hot.

Adjust portion sizes as needed to meet your individual dietary needs. You can also omit the cheese to reduce the fat content further.

103. Stuffed butternut squash with ground turkey and vegetables

Ingredient:

- 1 medium butternut squash, halved lengthwise and seeds removed
- 1 lb ground turkey
- 1 onion, diced
- 2 cloves garlic, minced
- 1 cup diced bell pepper
- 1 cup diced zucchini
- 1 tsp dried thyme
- 1 tsp dried oregano
- Salt and pepper to taste
- 1/4 cup shredded low•fat mozzarella cheese (optional)

Instructions:

1. Preheat oven to 400°F. Place the butternut squash halves cut•side up on a baking sheet. Bake for 40•50 minutes, until the squash is tender when pierced with a fork.

2. While the squash is baking, in a large skillet, cook the ground turkey over medium•high heat until browned and crumbled, about 5•7 minutes. Drain any excess fat.

3. Add the diced onion, garlic, bell pepper, and zucchini to the skillet. Sauté for 5•7 minutes until the vegetables are softened.

4. Stir in the dried thyme and oregano. Season with salt and pepper.

5. Once the squash is tender, scoop out the flesh, leaving about 1/2 inch of the squash intact to create a "boat". Mash the squash flesh and stir it into the turkey and vegetable mixture.

6. Spoon the turkey and vegetable stuffing back into the squash boats. If using, sprinkle the shredded mozzarella cheese over the top.

7. Return the stuffed squash halves to the oven and bake for an additional 10•15 minutes, until the cheese is melted. Serve hot.

Adjust portion sizes as needed to meet your individual dietary needs. You can also omit the cheese to reduce the fat content further.

104. Chicken and wild rice casserole

Ingredient:

- 1 lb boneless, skinless chicken breasts, diced
- 1 cup uncooked wild rice
- 2 cups low·sodium chicken broth
- 1 onion, diced
- 2 celery stalks, diced
- 1 cup sliced mushrooms
- 1 cup frozen peas
- 2 cloves garlic, minced
- 1 tsp dried thyme
- 1/2 tsp dried rosemary
- Salt and pepper to taste
- 1/4 cup shredded low·fat cheddar cheese (optional)

Instructions:

1. Preheat oven to 375°F. Spray a 9x13 inch baking dish with non·stick cooking spray.

2. In a medium saucepan, combine the wild rice and chicken broth. Bring to a boil, then reduce heat to low, cover, and simmer for 45·50 minutes, until rice is tender. Fluff with a fork.

3. In a large skillet, sauté the diced chicken over medium·high heat until cooked through, about 5·7 minutes. Remove chicken from skillet and set aside.

4. In the same skillet, sauté the diced onion, celery, and mushrooms for 5·7 minutes until softened. Add the minced garlic and sauté for 1 minute more.

5. In a large bowl, combine the cooked wild rice, sautéed chicken, vegetables, frozen peas, thyme, and rosemary. Season with salt and pepper.

6. Transfer the mixture to the prepared baking dish. If using, sprinkle the shredded cheese over the top.

7. Bake for 20·25 minutes, until heated through and cheese is melted.

8. Let stand for 5 minutes before serving.

Adjust portion sizes as needed to meet your individual dietary needs. You can also omit the cheese to reduce the fat content further.

105. Tuna and noodle casserole (with whole•grain noodles)

Ingredient:

• 8 oz whole•grain egg noodles
• 2 (5 oz) cans tuna, drained
• 1 cup frozen peas
• 1 cup low•fat milk
• 2 tbsp all•purpose flour
• 1 tsp dried thyme
• 1/2 tsp garlic powder
• 1/4 tsp black pepper
• 1/2 cup shredded low•fat cheddar cheese

Instructions:

1. Preheat oven to 375°F. Grease a 9x13 inch baking dish.

2. Cook the whole•grain egg noodles according to package instructions. Drain and set aside.

3. In a medium saucepan, whisk together the milk and flour over medium heat. Cook for 2•3 minutes, stirring constantly, until the mixture thickens.

4. Remove the saucepan from heat and stir in the dried thyme, garlic powder, and black pepper.

5. In a large bowl, combine the cooked noodles, drained tuna, frozen peas, and the milk•flour sauce. Mix well.

6. Transfer the tuna and noodle mixture to the prepared baking dish. Sprinkle the shredded cheddar cheese over the top.

7. Bake for 20•25 minutes, until the cheese is melted and bubbly. Let stand for 5 minutes before serving.

This tuna and whole•grain noodle casserole is a great option for those following a post•gastric bypass diet for several reasons:

• The whole•grain noodles provide fiber and complex carbs.
• The tuna is a lean protein source.
• The peas add additional fiber and nutrients.
• The reduced•fat cheese helps keep the dish lower in calories and fat.
• The casserole format makes it easy to portion and serve.

106. Turkey tetrazzini with whole•grain pasta

Ingredient:

• 8 oz whole•grain spaghetti or linguine, cooked al dente
• 1 lb ground turkey
• 1 onion, diced
• 2 cloves garlic, minced
• 8 oz sliced mushrooms
• 2 cups low•sodium chicken broth
• 1 cup low•fat milk
• 2 tbsp all•purpose flour
• 1 tsp dried thyme
• 1/2 tsp dried oregano
• Salt and pepper to taste
• 1/2 cup shredded low•fat mozzarella cheese

Instructions:
1. Preheat oven to 375°F. Grease a 9x13 inch baking dish.

2. In a large skillet, cook the ground turkey over medium•high heat until browned and crumbled, about 5•7 minutes. Drain any excess fat.

3. Add the diced onion and sliced mushrooms to the skillet. Sauté for 5•7 minutes until the vegetables are softened. Stir in the minced garlic and cook for 1 minute more.

4. In a small bowl, whisk together the chicken broth, milk, and flour until smooth. Pour this mixture into the skillet with the turkey and vegetables. Stir in the thyme, oregano, salt, and pepper.

5. Bring the sauce to a simmer and cook for 2•3 minutes, stirring constantly, until thickened.

6. Remove from heat and stir in the cooked whole•grain pasta.

7. Transfer the turkey tetrazzini mixture to the prepared baking dish. Sprinkle the shredded mozzarella cheese over the top.

8. Bake for 20•25 minutes, until the cheese is melted and bubbly. Let stand for 5 minutes before serving.

Adjust portion sizes as needed to meet your individual dietary needs. You can also use low•sodium broth and canned mushrooms to further reduce the sodium content.

107. Chicken pot pie with phyllo dough crust

Ingredient:

• 1 lb boneless, skinless chicken breasts, diced
• 2 cups low•sodium chicken broth
• 1 cup diced carrots
• 1 cup diced celery
• 1 cup diced onion
• 1 cup frozen peas
• 2 tbsp all•purpose flour
• 2 tbsp low•fat milk
• 1 tsp dried thyme
• Salt and pepper to taste

Crust Ingredients:
• 6 sheets phyllo dough, thawed if frozen
• 2 tbsp melted butter or olive oil

Instructions:
1. Preheat oven to 375°F.

2. In a large skillet, sauté the diced chicken over medium•high heat until cooked through, about 5•7 minutes. Remove chicken from skillet and set aside.

3. In the same skillet, sauté the carrots, celery, and onion for 5•7 minutes until softened.

4. Sprinkle the flour over the vegetable mixture and stir to coat. Gradually whisk in the chicken broth and milk. Bring to a simmer and cook for 2•3 minutes until thickened.

5. Stir the cooked chicken, peas, thyme, salt, and pepper into the vegetable mixture.

6. Spray a 9•inch pie dish with non•stick cooking spray. Layer 2 sheets of phyllo dough in the bottom and up the sides of the dish, brushing each layer with melted butter or oil.

7. Spoon the chicken and vegetable filling into the phyllo•lined dish.

8. Top with the remaining 4 sheets of phyllo dough, brushing each layer with melted butter or oil.

9. Bake for 30•35 minutes, until the phyllo crust is golden brown. Allow to cool for 5•10 minutes before serving.

108. Shepherd's pie with mashed cauliflower topping

Ingredient:

- 1 lb ground turkey or lean ground beef
- 1 onion, diced
- 2 carrots, peeled and diced
- 2 celery stalks, diced
- 2 cloves garlic, minced
- 1 tsp dried thyme
- 1 tsp dried rosemary
- 1 cup low•sodium beef or chicken broth
- 2 tbsp tomato paste
- Salt and pepper to taste

Topping Ingredients:
- 1 head of cauliflower, cut into florets
- 1/4 cup low•fat milk
- 2 tbsp grated Parmesan cheese
- Salt and pepper to taste

Instructions:

1. Preheat oven to 375°F. Grease a 9x13 inch baking dish.

2. In a large skillet, cook the ground turkey or beef over medium•high heat until browned and crumbled, about 5•7 minutes. Drain any excess fat.

3. Add the diced onion, carrots, celery, and garlic to the skillet. Sauté for 5•7 minutes until the vegetables are softened.

4. Stir in the dried thyme, rosemary, beef or chicken broth, and tomato paste. Season with salt and pepper.

5. Bring the mixture to a simmer and let it cook for 10•15 minutes, until the sauce has thickened.

6. Meanwhile, in a large pot, bring salted water to a boil. Add the cauliflower florets and cook until very tender, about 10•12 minutes. Drain the cauliflower and return it to the pot.

7. Add the milk to the cauliflower and mash with a potato masher or immersion blender until smooth and creamy. Stir in the Parmesan cheese and season with salt and pepper.

8. Spread the turkey or beef filling into the prepared baking dish. Top evenly with the mashed cauliflower.

9. Bake for 25•30 minutes, until the topping is lightly browned. Let stand for 5•10 minutes before serving.

109. Crustless spinach and feta quiche

Ingredient:

• 10 oz frozen chopped spinach, thawed and drained
• 6 large eggs
• 1 cup low•fat milk
• 1/2 tsp salt
• 1/4 tsp black pepper
• 1 cup crumbled feta cheese
• 2 tbsp grated Parmesan cheese

Instructions:

1. Preheat oven to 375°F. Grease a 9•inch pie dish with non•stick cooking spray.

2. Squeeze any excess moisture from the thawed spinach. Spread the spinach evenly in the prepared pie dish.

3. In a medium bowl, whisk together the eggs, milk, salt, and pepper until well combined.

4. Sprinkle the crumbled feta cheese over the spinach. Pour the egg mixture over the top.
5. Sprinkle the grated Parmesan cheese over the top of the quiche.

6. Bake for 35•40 minutes, until the center is set and the top is lightly golden.

7. Allow the quiche to cool for 5•10 minutes before slicing and serving.

This crustless spinach and feta quiche is a great option for those following a post•gastric bypass diet for several reasons:

• The eggs provide a good source of protein.
• The spinach adds fiber, vitamins, and minerals.
• The reduced•fat feta and Parmesan cheeses help keep the dish lower in calories and fat.
• The crustless format makes it easier to digest.

Adjust portion sizes as needed to meet your individual dietary needs. You can also experiment with other vegetable or cheese combinations.

Some tips for making this quiche post•gastric bypass friendly:
• Use low•fat or non•fat milk to reduce the fat content
• Avoid heavy cream or high•fat cheeses
• Stick to smaller portion sizes, as quiche can be rich
• Pair with a light salad or other low•calorie side dish

110. Crustless broccoli and cheddar quiche

Ingredient:

• 6 large eggs
• 1 cup low•fat milk
• 1/2 tsp salt
• 1/4 tsp black pepper
• 2 cups chopped broccoli florets
• 1 cup shredded low•fat cheddar cheese
• 2 tbsp grated Parmesan cheese

Instructions:

1. Preheat oven to 375°F. Grease a 9•inch pie dish with non•stick cooking spray.

2. In a large bowl, whisk together the eggs, milk, salt, and pepper until well combined.

3. Spread the chopped broccoli florets evenly in the prepared pie dish. Sprinkle the shredded cheddar cheese over the top.

4. Pour the egg mixture over the broccoli and cheese. Sprinkle the grated Parmesan cheese over the top.

5. Bake for 35•40 minutes, until the center is set and the top is lightly golden. Allow the quiche to cool for 5•10 minutes before slicing and serving.

This crustless broccoli and cheddar quiche is a great option for those following a post•gastric bypass diet for several reasons:

• The eggs provide a good source of protein.
• The broccoli adds fiber, vitamins, and minerals.
• The reduced•fat cheese helps keep the dish lower in calories and fat.
• The crustless format makes it easier to digest.

Adjust portion sizes as needed to meet your individual dietary needs. You can also experiment with other vegetable combinations or use different types of cheese.

Some tips for making this quiche post•gastric bypass friendly:
• Use low•fat or non•fat milk to reduce the fat content
• Avoid heavy cream or high•fat cheeses
• Stick to smaller portion sizes, as quiche can be rich
• Pair with a light salad or other low•calorie side dish

111. Baked apple with cinnamon

Ingredient:

- 4 medium•sized apples (such as Gala, Honeycrisp, or Fuji)
- 1/4 cup water
- 1 tsp ground cinnamon
- 1 tbsp honey (optional)

Instructions:

1. Preheat oven to 375°F. Lightly grease a baking dish or sheet.

2. Wash and core the apples, leaving a small well in the center of each one. Place the apples in the prepared baking dish.

3. Pour the water into the bottom of the baking dish.

4. Sprinkle the ground cinnamon evenly over the top of the apples. If using, drizzle the honey over the apples as well.

5. Bake for 30•40 minutes, until the apples are tender when pierced with a fork.

6. Remove the baked apples from the oven and let cool for 5 minutes before serving.

This baked apple with cinnamon is a great dessert option for those following a post•gastric bypass diet for several reasons:

- Apples are a low•calorie, high•fiber fruit that can help satisfy sweet cravings.
- Cinnamon adds flavor without any added sugar.
- The honey (if using) provides a touch of sweetness without a lot of added sugar.
- The baked format is easy to digest.

Adjust portion sizes as needed to meet your individual dietary needs. You can also experiment with different spice combinations, such as adding a pinch of nutmeg or ginger.

Some tips for making this post•gastric bypass friendly:
- Use small to medium•sized apples
- Avoid adding too much honey or other sweeteners
- Pair with a small serving of plain Greek yogurt for added protein
- Stick to one baked apple per serving

112. Grilled peaches with yogurt

Ingredient:

• 4 ripe but firm peaches, halved and pitted
• 1 tbsp olive oil or coconut oil
• 1 cup plain Greek yogurt
• 2 tbsp honey (optional)
• 1 tsp vanilla extract
• Chopped fresh mint or basil for garnish (optional)

Instructions:

1. Preheat grill or grill pan to medium·high heat.

2. Brush the cut sides of the peach halves with the oil.

3. Place the peach halves cut·side down on the grill and cook for 3·5 minutes, until grill marks appear and the peaches are slightly softened.

4. Carefully flip the peach halves and grill for an additional 2·3 minutes.

5. Remove the grilled peaches from the grill and let cool slightly.

6. In a small bowl, mix together the Greek yogurt, honey (if using), and vanilla extract.

7. Place the grilled peach halves on a serving plate or individual plates. Top each peach half with a dollop of the yogurt mixture.

8. Garnish with chopped fresh mint or basil, if desired. Serve immediately.

This grilled peaches with yogurt dessert is a great option for those following a post·gastric bypass diet for several reasons:

• Peaches are a low·calorie, high·fiber fruit that can help satisfy sweet cravings.
• Greek yogurt provides protein and probiotics to support gut health.
• The honey (if using) adds a touch of sweetness without a lot of added sugar.
• The dish is light, refreshing, and easy to digest.

Adjust portion sizes as needed to meet your individual dietary needs. You can also experiment with different fruit and yogurt flavor combinations.

113. Frozen yogurt bark with berries

Ingredient:

- 2 cups plain Greek yogurt
- 2 tbsp honey (optional)
- 1 tsp vanilla extract
- 1 cup mixed berries (such as blueberries, raspberries, and/or blackberries)

Instructions:

1. Line a baking sheet with parchment paper or a silicone baking mat.

2. In a medium bowl, mix together the Greek yogurt, honey (if using), and vanilla extract until well combined.

3. Spread the yogurt mixture evenly onto the prepared baking sheet, creating a thin, even layer.

4. Sprinkle the mixed berries evenly over the top of the yogurt.

5. Place the baking sheet in the freezer and freeze for at least 2•3 hours, or until the yogurt bark is completely frozen.

6. Once frozen, break or cut the yogurt bark into pieces and serve immediately. Store any leftover pieces in an airtight container in the freezer.

This frozen yogurt bark with berries is a great option for those following a post•gastric bypass diet for several reasons:

- The Greek yogurt provides protein and probiotics.
- The berries add fiber, vitamins, and antioxidants.
- The honey (if using) provides a touch of sweetness without a lot of added sugar.
- The frozen format makes it a refreshing and satisfying dessert or snack.
- The portion•controlled pieces make it easy to enjoy in moderation.

Adjust the amount of honey used or omit it entirely to further reduce the sugar content if desired. You can also experiment with different fruit combinations.

Some tips for making this post•gastric bypass friendly:
- Use plain, unsweetened Greek yogurt
- Avoid high•fat toppings or mix•ins
- Stick to smaller portion sizes, as frozen treats can be filling
- Pair with a light meal or as a standalone snack

Congratulations on reaching the end of ***"The Post-Gastric Bypass Cookbook: 110+ Nutritious Recipes for Post-Gastric Bypass Success."*** By exploring these recipes and integrating them into your daily routine, you have taken significant steps towards ensuring a healthy and fulfilling post-surgery life.

Reflecting on Your Journey

Gastric bypass surgery is a powerful tool for weight loss and improved health, but it is your commitment to making sustainable lifestyle changes that will ultimately determine your success. This cookbook has been designed to support you every step of the way, providing you with delicious, nutritious, and easy-to-prepare meals that cater to your specific needs.

Celebrating Your Progress

As you continue on your journey, take a moment to celebrate your progress. Each meal you prepare and enjoy from this book is a testament to your dedication and resilience. Remember, the changes you make in the kitchen extend far beyond your plate; they impact your overall well-being, energy levels, and quality of life.

Staying Inspired and Informed

The road to a healthier you is ongoing. Stay inspired by revisiting these recipes, experimenting with new ingredients, and continually educating yourself about nutrition and healthy eating habits. Join support groups, consult with your healthcare providers, and stay connected with others who share your journey.

Your Support System

Remember that you are not alone. Your healthcare team, family, and friends are valuable sources of support. Lean on them when you need encouragement, and don't hesitate to seek professional guidance if you encounter challenges.

Thank you for allowing "The Post-Gastric Bypass Cookbook: 110+ Nutritious Recipes for Post-Gastric Bypass Success" to be a part of your journey. We hope that these recipes have inspired you and equipped you with the tools you need to thrive. Here's to your continued success, health, and culinary adventures.

Bon Appétit and Best Wishes!

With warmest regards,